SEX ENERGY
&
ORGASMIC ECSTASY

Realize Your Full Sexual Potential
&
Transform it into Pure Joy

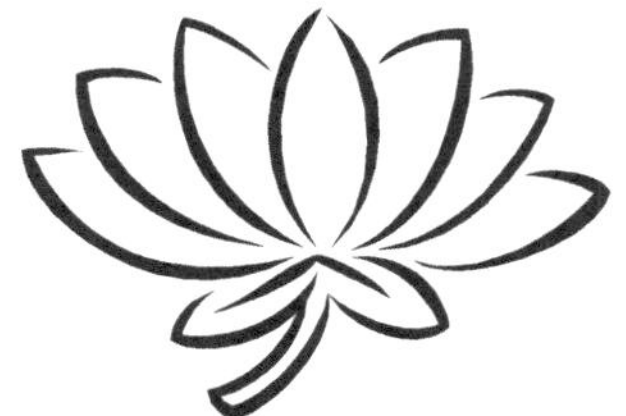

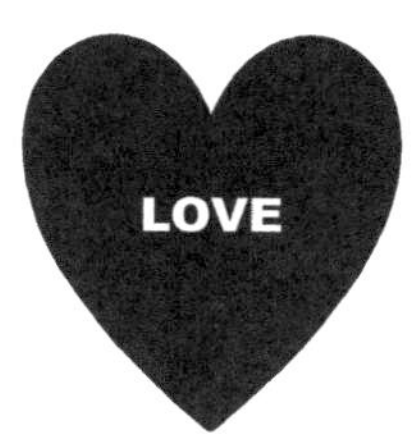

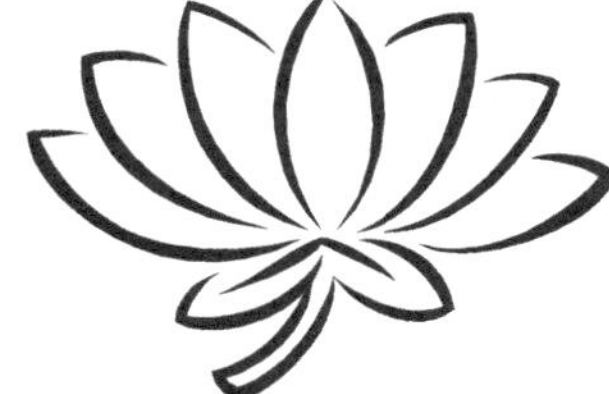

SACHIN J. KARNIK, Ph.D.

LCSW, LCDP, CAADC, ICGC-II/BACC, CPS

SEX ENERGY & ORGASMIC ECSTASY

 For more information about the ideas discussed in this book, please contact the author at: sachinkarnik@yahoo.com.

ISBN-13: 978-1979421959
ISBN-10: 1979421951

WARNING: ADULT MATERIAL.

There are techniques discussed in this book on human sexuality. This book does not give any psychiatric, psychological or other diagnoses or and suggestions for medications. If you have a medical condition, a medical doctor should be consulted. People who have high blood pressure, heart disease, or a generally weak condition should consult their doctor before engaging in any of the techniques shown in this book. The techniques discussed in this book are an extract from various traditions that combine meditation with sex stimulation.

To order additional copies of this book, please visit:

Amazon.com
Create Space E-Stores at createspace.com

or contact the author at:

sachinkarnik@yahoo.com
Smart Phone: 302-650-3865
Please leave your name and phone number and the author will contact you. You may also send text messages.

Published by: Sachin Karnik
Distributed by: createspace.com

DEDICATION

This book is dedicated to you, the reader.
May you uncover amazing truths about sex energy and immerse yourself in pure and undisturbed happiness.

TABLE OF CONTENTS

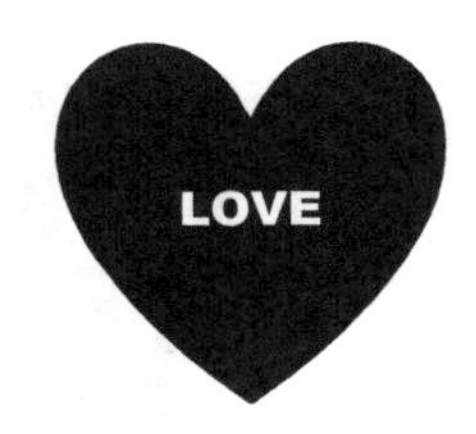

CHAPTER 2
OVERVIEW OF SEXUAL RESPONSE

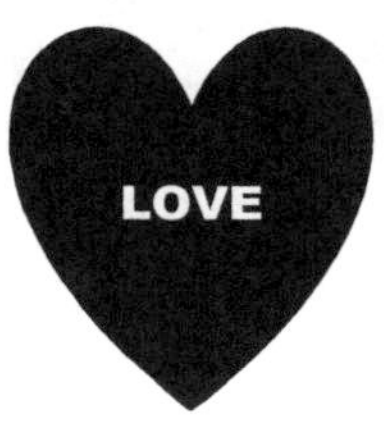

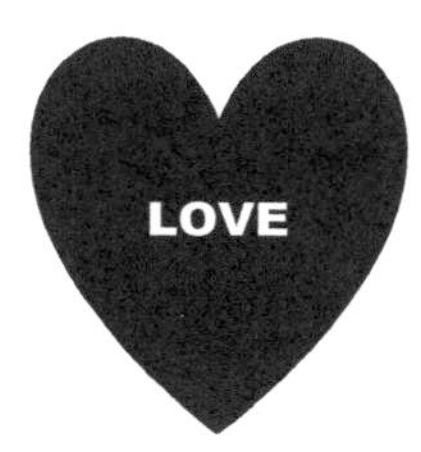

CHAPTER 3
EJACULATORY ORGASMS, POINT OF NO RETURN, & MEDITATIVE SEXUAL PRACTICES

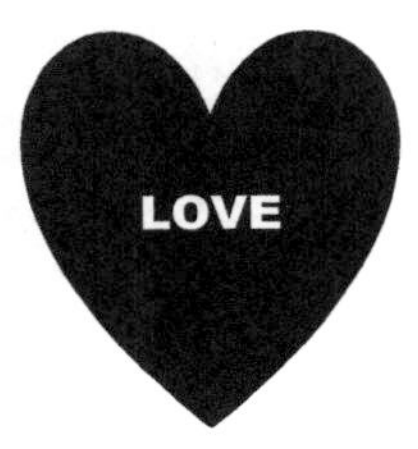

CHAPTER 4
CONTROL OF SEXUAL ENERGY

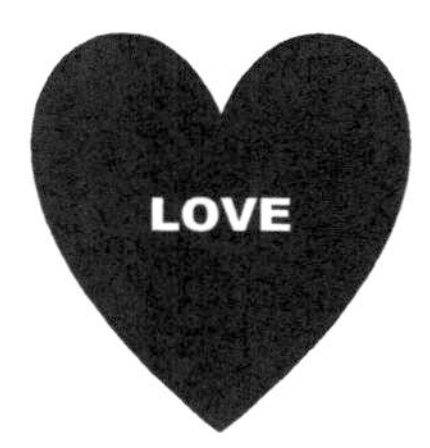

CHAPTER 5
MIND, SEX ENERGY& PSYCHOLOGICAL FRAGMENTATION

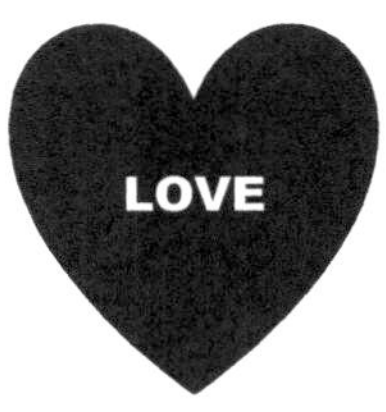

CHAPTER 6
MEDITATION & SEX ENERGY TRANSMUTATION

CHAPTER 7
ORGASMIC ENERGY &
SEX ENERGY TRANSMUTATION VIA PRE-ORGASMIC SEXUAL PRACTICES

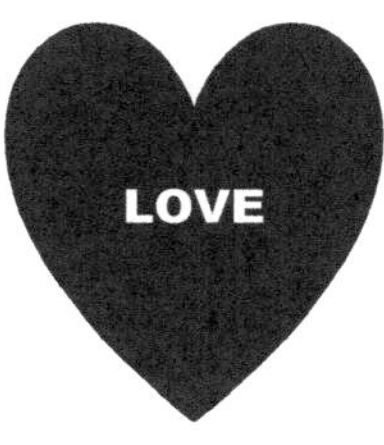

Chapter 7: Continued....

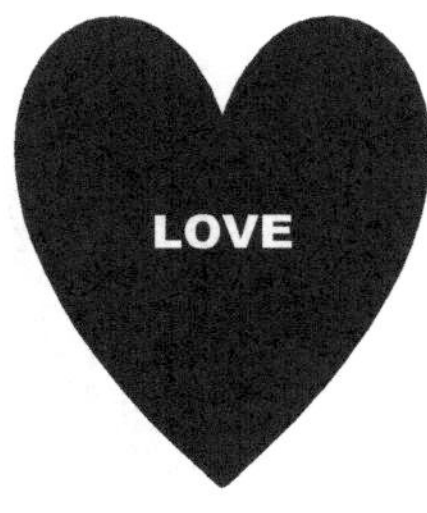

Chapter 7: Continued....

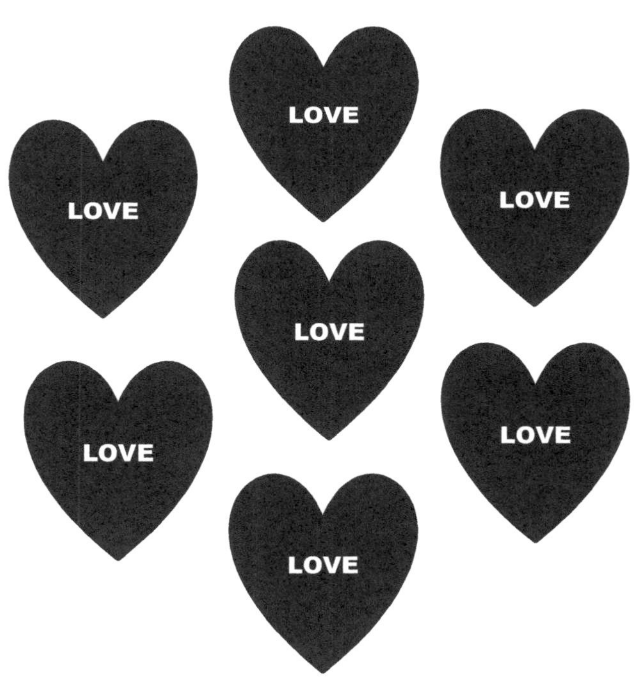

CHAPTER 8
SEX & RELATIONSHIPS

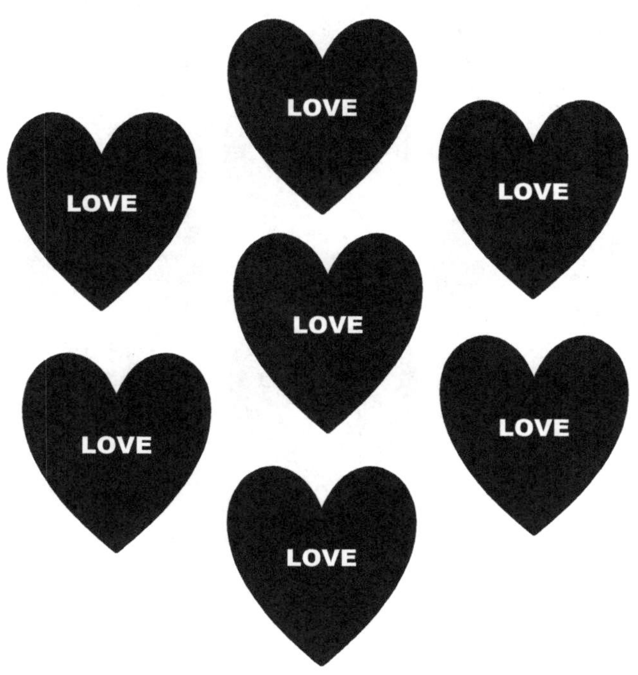

CHAPTER 9
ECSTATIC LIVING & THE INWARD JOURNEY

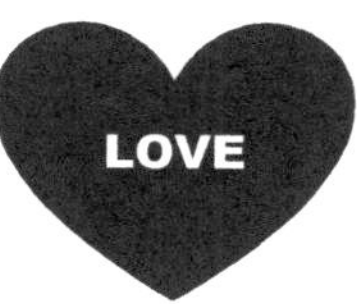

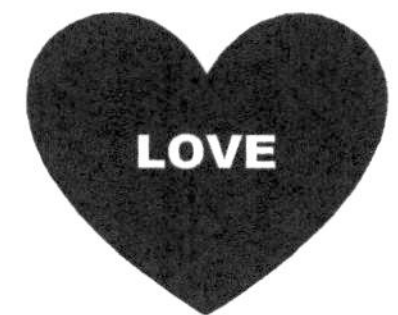

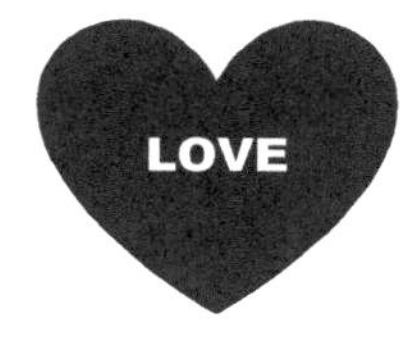

THE "HEART" & THREE MEDITATIONS AT THE BEGINNING

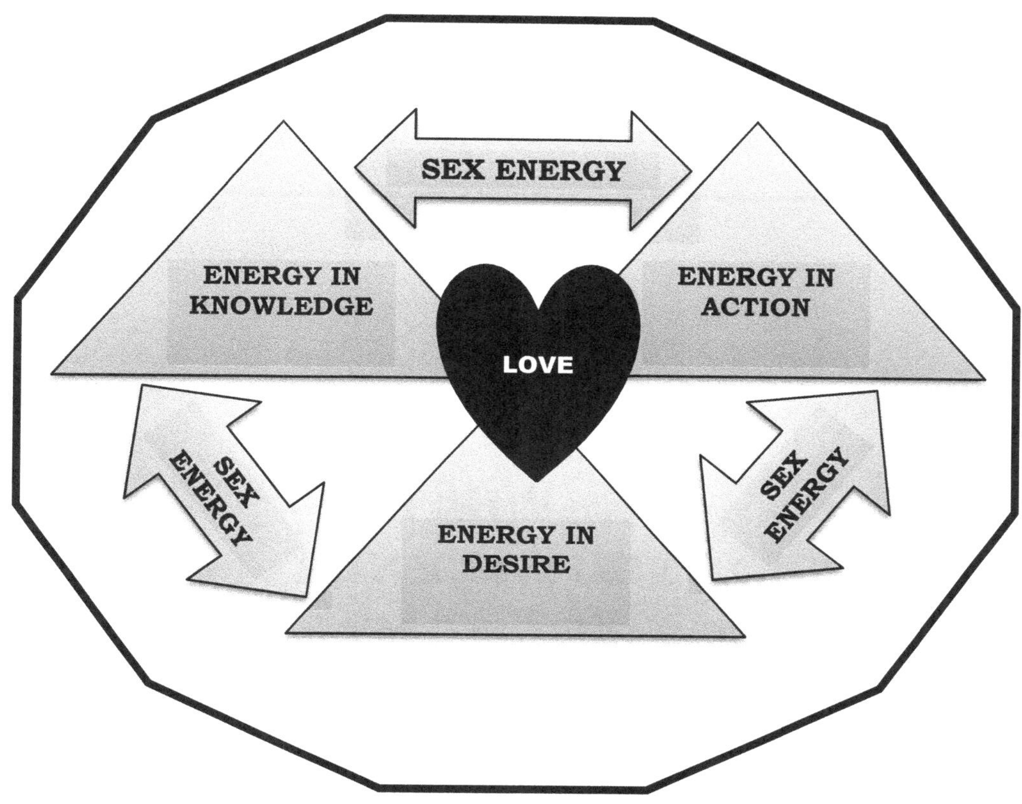

You are pure love. This love exists within the center of your own being where energies combine. The figure above is a dodecagon (12-sided figure) that represents 12 areas of one's life that *will* function in a highly integrated way when energies existing in knowledge, desire, and action combines together. These energies are aspects of one's raw sex energy that can transform and opens the doorway into pure, undiluted love. The 12 areas of one's life are:

1) Love Relationship
2) Friendships
3) Adventures
4) Environment
5) Health & Fitness
6) Intellectual Life
7) Your Skills
8) Spiritual Life
9) Career
10) Creative Life
11) Family Life
12) Community Life

MEDITATION # 1

Find a quiet place to sit.
Read the question below.
Close your eyes and visualize the question.
Hold the words in your mind and heart.
Notice what you are thinking and feeling with your eyes closed.

WHAT
TRUTHS EXIST
ABOUT MY
SEX LIFE THAT
ONLY I KNOW?

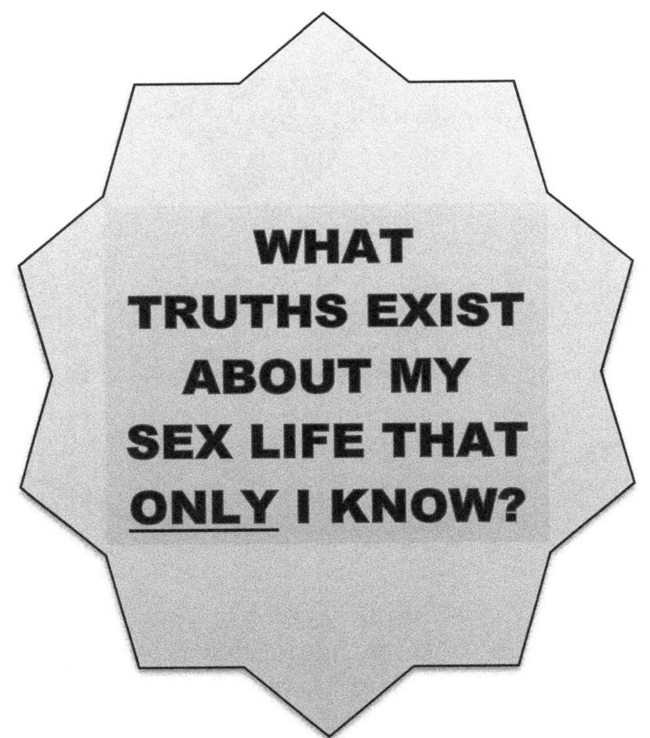

MEDITATION # 2

Find a quiet place to sit.
Read the question below.
Close your eyes and visualize the question.
Hold the words in your mind and heart.
Notice what you are thinking and feeling with your eyes closed.

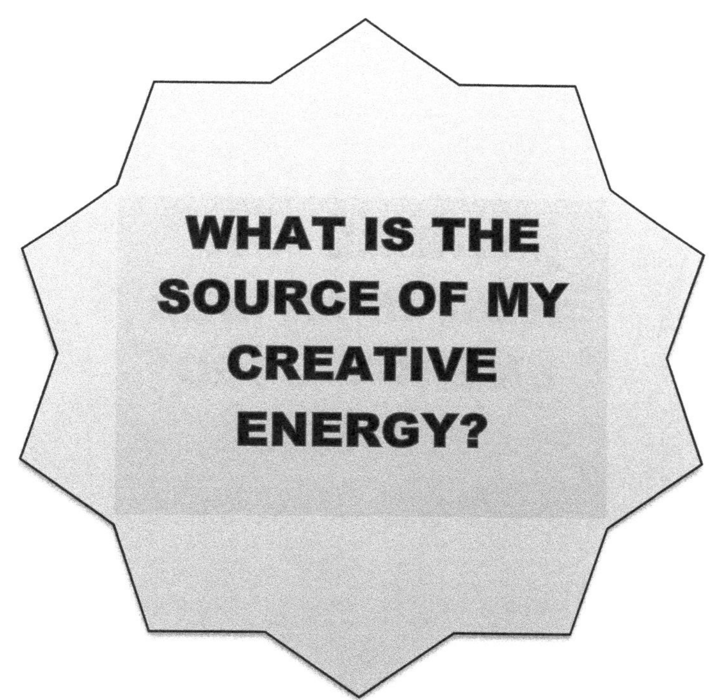

MEDITATION # 3

Find a quiet place to sit.
Read the question below.
Close your eyes and visualize the question.
Hold the words in your mind and heart.
Notice what you are thinking and feeling with your eyes closed.

WHERE AND HOW IS MY SEX ENERGY USED?

There is only ONE energy that takes innumerable forms. Sex energy is one's root energy that originates in the cosmos.

-- Sachin J. Karnik

PREFACE

Welcome friends to a fantastic exploration of sex. As humans are explorers by nature, this book is an exploratory journey into unravel amazing truths about sex and sex energy. The power to write these words comes from energy and your power to read these words comes from the same energy. This may seem strange or unusual somehow, yet it is profoundly true because sex energy is *the* root energy within each human being. The experience of sex and the pleasures inherent within it are truly nonverbal. When one is intensely absorbed in sexual enjoyment, there are really no words because the experience is beyond language. Furthermore, the mind's disturbances are significantly diminished (temporarily) when one is in a state of euphoria. The question then becomes: "Is it possible to live in a state where all psychological disturbances have stopped and only a constant state of pure, non-diluted, non-fragmented, whole bliss abides?" In this journey of exploring sexual energy and pleasure, the hope is to discover profound truths about sexuality, the pursuit of pleasure, and possibly, the soul's journey toward the Divine. (**Please note that in this book, the word "Divine" is used to mean: God, the soul, the spirit beyond matter, the spiritual dimension of one's being, a higher conscious state, the transcendental state of realization, and/or the solidification of truth-bliss-consciousness.)

There is no doubt that you picked up this book because a part of you is curious to know about the connection between sex energy and pleasure. The use of energy to create the experience of pleasure is centrally explored in this book. In the opinion of the author, disturbances in one's sex energy create a human existence filled with internal conflicts that will have profound consequences in multiple areas of life. In fact, it is the author's contention that, throughout the world, there is a significant lack of awareness about the relationship between orgasms, erotic pleasures, ecstatic pleasure and the nature of energy within the body and the mind. A major goal in this book is to show a possible synthesis of these aspects of sexuality - to take a journey into the unfolding of inner truth, in which the energy required to create unity among these aspects actually causes that unity to flower from within.

Of course, this book can also be used to gain greater conceptual understanding about sexual energies and their relationship to a spiritual dimension in one's being. This may be a great starting point if one has never considered how to combine sexual stimulation with meditation. At its core, the theme of this book is about increasing awareness that each person has a reservoir of massive energy within himself/herself and most importantly, it is possible to learn how to use that reservoir to accomplish worldly and spiritual goals. This book aims to provide a powerful conceptual understanding of the connection between orgasm, meditation, and spiritual development. If one chooses to practice techniques that bring about this connection, one will gain first-hand experience of the connection. Such a state of connection will be one beyond the limits of any language to express.

If one is following a strict traditional spiritual path that dictates strict vows of celibacy or limited sexual activity, then this book will certainly give the reader a unique perspective on the relationship between pleasure and the Divine. Of course, some readers may not choose to practice techniques that combine sexual pleasures with meditation; nonetheless, there are a multitude of ideas that could potentially give one great insight into making progress on one's chosen path. In the author's opinion, the reality of sex is the *one thing* from which there is no escape, irrespective of one's spiritual path. Therefore, this book discusses some traditional paths that promote control of sex energy where sex sublimation is sought after through control of desire. This has been termed as a "**Warrior's Path**."

The author suspects, however, that many who have picked up this book have strong sexual desires and deep sexual intensity whether one is religious/spiritual or not. This book is written especially for those who are deeply sexual and want to experience greater, enhanced, and more intense sexual pleasure with transformative potential. For all readers with deep-seated sexual desires (most of the adult human population), this book proposes the idea that sex is not one's enemy in making progress in meditation or even spiritual (inward) growth.

Many highly sexual people feel that their sexuality prevents them from progressing further spiritually (inwardly). One's sexuality *is* one's intensity. Intense sexuality is erotic and the various meditation techniques shown will illustrate how to infuse meditation into erotic sexuality and turn it into ecstasy. Such a state of ecstasy, has within it, great love pouring out for *all* of creation. Transformation from "erotic" to "ecstatic" is a wondrous result of combining meditation with sexual stimulation.

Although many books already exist in the market regarding "tantric sex, sacred sex, multi-orgasmic sex, etc.," these books, in the author's opinion, *do not give to the general public at large*, the type of intelligibility required to actually connect orgasmic pleasures with subtle dimensions of one's being. Although reading such books can be helpful in providing multiple perspectives on sex and orgasms, this book can serve as a great foundation in understanding and accepting some hard to believe facts such as:

- Orgasm and ejaculation are separate processes (for men).
- Orgasm and ejaculation can be separated by specific techniques (for men).

- Orgasmic energy can be cultivated and used to enhance physical health, mental health, emotional healing, and spiritual awakening.
- It is possible to experience a state of ecstasy that touches the spiritual dimension within by allowing orgasmic energies to flow throughout the body.

The fact is that any book, including this one, can only point out certain truths. ***It will be up to you (the reader) to see the reality of what is written for yourself***. Only then one will develop deep awareness that sexual pleasures and psycho-spiritual development are not contradictory. They are complementary, in which the most intense orgasm is merely a fragment of the bliss of pure consciousness. It is the author's sincere, heartfelt optimism that, if one chooses to experiment with sex meditation techniques, it will be done with sincerity, patience, and open-mindedness. The techniques shown can be used in various modes of sexual stimulation: 1) solo-masturbation mode, 2) sexual intimacy with partner, and 3) other modes as one sees fit. A sincere attempt has been made to lay a solid conceptual foundation upon which actual practices of meditative sex are based. These practices are extremely powerful and potent. Even the slightest progress made using these practices can be felt within one's life in the form of increased energy, deeper understanding, and growing love. It is the author's sincere wish that you (the reader) will make every effort to look within yourself and try your best to become aware of the multitude of psycho-sexual processes that are occurring within you. If one does not do this, then at best, only a conceptual understanding will be gained. The real power of this book can be experienced through **introspection** (i.e. looking within) and experimenting with the movements of sexual desires within oneself.

With regards to the text, you will see words that have been bolded. Each **bold word** or **bold phrase** is defined in the glossary section for your reference. The entire book is inter-connected with interlocking concepts. The glossary section can be used as a quick reference in understanding various terms and concepts. Please also make special note that concepts, ideas, and techniques discussed in this book are written in language of heterosexuality, they are equally applicable to the **LBGTQ** population. Also, there are 12 contemplative diagrams for self-reflection and discussion.

If you have any comments or questions regarding the material presented, please contact me via e-mail at: sachinkarnik@yahoo.com or call me at: 302-650-3865. My full contact information is written at the end of the book. To order additional copies of this book at a discounted rate, please contact me directly.

CHAPTER 1

INTRODUCTION

LET THE JOURNEY BEGIN!

Human behavior flows from three main sources: desire, emotion, and knowledge.

--Plato[A]

SEX! SEX! & MORE SEX!!!

The entire world is in relentless pursuit of sexual pleasures. It is truly astounding when one considers how much time, energy, and money drives the pursuit, repetition, and enhancement of sexual pleasures. Undoubtedly, sex is one of the greatest mysteries in life and an extraordinary personal experience. For millennia, humans have probed into and experimented with sex as it continues to remain an unfathomable mystery. Indisputably, we all have an inborn (instinctual) need to experience sexual pleasure. Humans have discovered countless ways over thousands of years to enhance sexual pleasures. In fact, a great portion of each person's life is devoted to finding methods and means of experiencing sexual pleasures, satisfying sexual appetites fully, and further enhancing orgasmic experiences. This pursuit of orgasmic pleasure is deeply embedded in the minds of the human population living on our beautiful planet. If one accepts this, one must also accept the fact that human intelligence has the capability to examine the magnificence of sex. We are the only species that has the aptitude to study, enhance, and examine in multiple ways the nature of our sexuality. This investigation/examination is of two types:

Subjective Examination: This examination is one's *personal and intimate* experience of sex. This means that one knows, *within one's inner depths*, the actual potency and pleasure experienced in sexual stimulation. Examining sex subjectively demands looking at one's own experience of sex *as it is* without distortion. Clear awareness of personal sexual experiences can provide profound intuitive (inner) understanding and personal transformation.

Objective Examination: Examining sex objectively refers to unfolding and studying a multitude of neurobiological processes by scientific methods, as has been done by many scientific disciplines. In studying the biology of sex, one would find an elaborate description of the anatomy and physiology of sexual organs and complex arrays of biochemical processes.

Given these two ways of understanding sex, a subjective examination of sexuality is a different matter altogether from sheer objective or factual scientific knowledge about anatomy and physiology. A subjective examination is an explorative journey into the nature of *one's own* mind and its role in the entire sexual process. The human mind is one of the greatest mysteries in the universe given its subtlety, speed, and powers. In each human being, there are varying degrees of awareness of emotions, thoughts, feelings, and memories. There exists the capacity to create change within the mind by using energy intelligently and utilizing one's decision-making ability for one's benefit.

Humanity has an intrinsic capacity to explore the inner world of thoughts, emotions, memories and desires. As a psychotherapist and spiritual seeker, the writer has studied sexuality and particularly have studied the role of sex energy in spiritual transformation. During this 20 years of study, many remarkable and extraordinary truths about sex energy have been revealed. The intention in writing this book is to open multiple dimensions of sexual experiences, and the role of these experiences in potentially unlocking greater happiness and joy within each person. Each person is in pursuit of joy, happiness, pleasure, well-being, healthy relationships, etc. In this pursuit, sexual pleasure certainly has a prominent place.

Potent experiences provided by sexual stimulation are deeply sought after for at least two basic reasons:

1) *Sex feels very, very good…*given that a concentrated and compelling experience of pleasure occurs.
2) Sex is the means for reproduction and humanity's survival depends on it.

Nature has linked procreation with intense pleasure to ensure unbroken continuation and survival of humanity. Given that sexual drive is deeply instinctual, and humanity owes its existence to it, it is an incontrovertible truth that quite a bit of time, effort, and energy (physical & mental) is expended in the pursuit of repeated sexual gratification. Starting in adolescence and continuing into adulthood, each person dedicates a substantial proportion of thought, energy, time, money, etc. in pursuing and ultimately experiencing repeated cycles of sexual pleasure. One must pay homage to this great creative power given that each person's existence is due to this power. In fact, the entire physical body is a corporeal manifestation of sex energy, and hence, it is a sex energy phenomenon. There is *one* fundamental energy flowing through the entire neuropsychological system and expressing itself within each person's emotions, thoughts, memories and desires, along with countless other **neurophysiological** and **neuropsychological** processes. In other words, without the presence of **sexual energy** (i.e. fundamental core energy in the brain and spinal cord), there would be absolutely no mental or physical function. Hence, there would be no life. Life as we know it is a manifestation of this highly potent, creative power this is experienced as "**sex energy**." In fact, many spiritual traditions have referred to sex energy as the "power of God." The demand for sexual gratification is one of the deepest cravings that resides in the heart of each human being, due to its life-giving potential. The *power of sex* and the *power within sex* cannot be taken lightly, because this power can be utilized to develop and enhance physical, psychological, and spiritual strength. When this power is utilized for destructive rather than constructive purposes, it can place one in great misery due to lacking awareness of the importance of cultivating and transforming sex energy in a positive direction. The lack of cultivation of sex energy causes, in the opinion of the author, great misery for millions of human beings. Problems ranging from relationship issues between couples to over-population problems have their roots in the lack of adequate **sublimation** (not **suppression**) of sexual energies and **sexual essences**.

TARGET AUDIENCE OF THIS BOOK

Who is the target audience for this book? The target audience consists of 5 diverse groups:

a) ***This book is for all men*** who would like to learn about harnessing their sexual potential beyond just **ejaculatory orgasms**.

b) ***This book is for all women*** who are seeking multiple orgasms with their partners. Many women are sexually frustrated due to their male partners not paying enough attention to their needs. Deeper orgasmic connection between partners is vital in the overall development of a relationship.

c) ***This book is for spiritually minded people*** who are keenly interested in knowing how **sex energy sublimation** and spiritual development are connected. Learning non-sexual techniques of sex sublimation can provide a good foundation for further spiritual development. Many sincere spiritual seekers have serious issues with their sexuality and are in a state of conflict within themselves due to sexual desires pulling them on one side and, on the other hand, desire for real spiritual development (i.e. God realization, Self-Realization, **Nirvana**, **Heaven**, **Moksha**, etc.) There is currently and has been historically, a serious split in the personality of many spiritual aspirants with regards to sex. There are many techniques of sex sublimation that emphasize control of sexual impulses using non-sexual methods of meditation. The limitations of control and the various problems created by attempting to control powerful sexual impulses are also discussed to show how sexual energies can be sublimated naturally without the need for a psychological war with sexual desires. The intention is to examine the nature of self-imposed control vs. natural control. Natural control does not have the major problem of psychological warfare with one's own deep-seated sexual desires. Many of these control-oriented approaches are present, in some form or another, in a multitude of spiritual and/or religious paths throughout the world. Essential concepts have been extracted and have been presented in a very applicable and straightforward manner, so that anyone interested in truly becoming established in a state of absolute sex energy sublimation (**brahmacharya**, also known as the **urdhva-reeta** state) can find applicable and interesting ideas.

d) ***This book is for students and teachers of sexuality.*** This book can be extremely helpful in supplementing foundational textbooks on human sexuality. If one is interested in using this book as a supplement to more scientifically oriented textbooks on human sexuality, then studying this book in its entirety is strongly recommended. This book gives specific techniques to achieve male multiple-whole-body orgasms without ejaculation. Many students and their teachers will be interested to know how this is achieved. Although there are many books available on **tantric sex** and **sacred sex**, etc., *this* book aims to bring greater clarity to these topics by presenting a more integrated view of the flow of sex energy.

e) ***This book, of course, is for all of humanity.*** Humanity is psychologically stuck with painful conflicts in all dimensions of life. Unquestionably, there is a necessity in everyone's life to increase joy and find reasonable/meaningful solutions to serious problems. With humility, it is the writer's contention that true flowering of sexual power within each person can greatly reduce and possibly eliminate, at the root, all psychological conflict. Anyone living in such an extraordinary state *will* generate positive repercussions within multiple layers of society. The fact is, sex energy is an intensely profound experiential reality in each person's life, and to understand it, embrace it, and transform it is the birthright of every human being. Such profound transformation can unlock deeply hidden truths within each person leading to a state of complete harmony and unbounded bliss in all dimensions of life. This statement is made from a viewpoint that each human being has the birthright to tap into an infinite reservoir of happiness that remains hidden. In most people, pure and undiluted joy remain covered. ***Pleasure* moves in a wave, with peaks and valleys, on the substratum of absolute joy.** Realization of this truth is a matter of direct and personal acceptance of joy not merely being a conceptual construct. Opening the fountain of pure and undiluted happiness (joy or **ananda**) is possible for each person who goes through transformation. Just as a caterpillar becomes a butterfly, an ordinary human being can become a transformed individual where creative energy is unlocked from within. A butterfly is colorful, has wings, and can fly. It never reverts to its former life of becoming a caterpillar. This is the main difference between change and transformation. Change in life is like a caterpillar moving from one point to another. Transformation is comparable to a caterpillar becoming a butterfly. Most of humanity is stuck in mere change and does not know the glory of transformation. Sexual energy can awaken and transform into highly refined forms while the substratum of pure joy can be realized without being at war with orgasmic pleasure. Orgasmic pleasure is comparable to waves on the ocean, while pure joy (**ananda**) is the ocean itself. The wave is nothing but the ocean in a different form. Similarly, orgasmic pleasure is another form of joy, and it owes its existence to the substratum of pure joy.

IS SEX MERELY A TENSION RELIEVER?

As stated before, this book is written for both men and women. Emphasis on male sexuality has been placed in several sections of this book, because many men are not aware that transformation of **sexual essences** is possible by mixing meditation with sexual stimulation. Men can develop their sexuality further to make multiple whole-body orgasms possible. For many men, the concept of multiple orgasms or whole-body orgasms seems fanciful because there is a primeval psychological fixation in each man's mind to ejaculate into a women's vagina. Due to this fixation, most men do not know that there are other delightful possibilities for their sex energy that go beyond the limited yet explosive experience of **genital orgasm**. It is possible for men to become aware of the limitations of genital orgasm by becoming masters of their own sexual energy. Such mastery is possible by combining meditation with sexual stimulation.

Women reading this book will be able to assist their male sexual partner in mastering many techniques shown in this book. In fact, if you are a woman and have a male sexual partner, it is *imperative* that you read this book as it can enhance your relationship and bring greater sexual satisfaction and fulfillment to you. One of the major problems in sexual relations between partners is that sex has become a very limited act that lasts anywhere from 5 minutes to 15 minutes because many men reach their climax point long before their female partners have had at least one orgasm. This causes a multitude of problems for couples due to two basic reasons:

1) Many men use sex as a "tension reliever" and do not know exactly how to engage in the sex act in a meditative way to foster a deeper connection with their partner.

2) Women who do not experience a full orgasm remain frustrated, and this causes arguments, loneliness, extra-marital affairs, anger, and at times, even divorce.

Women can have multiple orgasms, and many men are not cognizant about the great sexual and orgasmic potential that resides within their female partner. Men can develop great respect for their female partner by first being concerned with helping her achieve multiple orgasms. Female orgasms are essential in the development of robust physical and emotional connections between partners. Consequently, the practices shown for men in this book will benefit women extensively *if* they take an active role in assisting their male partner in harnessing his sexual power. In most cases, men are seeking **genital orgasm** (which is a limited act) and this can result in depletion of energy. Relaxation experienced after ejaculating is a type of "**negative relaxation**" and generally causes a state of low energy. Heavy losses of this sexual energy can potentially have serious physical and mental health consequences if an obsession with genital orgasm occurs.[1]

Genital orgasm has become, for countless men, a means of temporary stress and tension reduction. Certainly, having occasional ejaculatory orgasms is quite natural and healthy as they are peak experiences in the human sexual pleasure cycle. Nonetheless, please consider the possibility that a copious amount of energy is utilized in ejaculatory orgasms, causing significant loss of potent sexual power where this power (energy) has the possibility of being stored in a refined form in the mind. (This statement is being made in a general sense and may not be applicable to all men. There are many factors that determine the level of loss of energy, and it is up to everyone to make a personal assessment as to how much energy is lost and the resulting effects of the lost energy. It is a biological fact that a great amount of energy is used by the brain and other organs to produce the experience of an ejaculatory orgasm.) The intention of the author is to give a powerful alternative where ***sex stimulation can be very enjoyable without significant depletion of energy,*** with the potential of reducing/eliminating stress and tension within deeper layers of the mind. This is possible through cultivation of sexual essences using **pre-orgasmic mini-currents**. The actual meditation techniques for this are covered in chapter 7. Suffice it to say, at this juncture, that a true flowering of male and female sexuality can potentially occur due to synchronous orgasmic balancing between partners. Women can have multiple orgasms, and it behooves the male partner to ensure that this occurs. Many men are deeply fixated on reaching sexual climax quickly, missing completely many wonderful opportunities and possibilities for harnessing their own energy. They may forget (while being absorbed in their own desire to reach sexual climax) that they are engaged in the sex act to activate pleasure within their partner. Therefore, the ideas, truths, and practices shown in this book are for both men and women so that greater awareness of sexual energies can take place and bring about sustained joy and well-being.

Please note that, in addition to readers interested in relationship development, this book is for those who wish to understand the connection between orgasms and ecstatic spirituality. This may seem contradictory, yet, in the opinion of the writer, there is a great relationship between spiritual development and orgasmic energy. This has been described in chapter 3 as the "**Sex-Orgasm-Celibacy Continuum**."

> ***During orgasmic states, the disturbances of the mind are significantly reduced or even stopped. This is a glimpse of a permanent state beyond all disturbance. Concentration of sex energy creates orgasmic peaks. Orgasms cannot exist without intense energy.***
>
> ***-- Sachin J. Karnik***

THE MYSTERY OF SEXUAL ATTRACTION (The Sexual Urge)

Sexual urges are inherently present biologically and psychologically in every human being. Each of us goes through **puberty** (phase of development that begins the sexual processes in boys and girls), and we eventually mature as fully sexual adults. Complex biological processes of sexual maturation are programmed in the human **genome** for the purpose of reproduction. This process is so intricate, that along with numerous physical changes during puberty, intensification of sexual desire begins to occur during adolescence. Sexual exploration begins in adolescence and grows into sexual appetites as adolescence transitions into adulthood. During adolescence and then into adulthood, the psychological need for sexual pleasure places enormous pressure on an individual to fulfill sexual urges and sexual appetites. As adolescents and many pre-adolescents become increasingly familiar with their sexual organs, their initial experiences of sexual pleasure occur. These experiences may be part of personal relationships via dating or other modalities where many adolescents begin sexual activity. **Infatuation** with the opposite sex may also occur, leading to a variety of emotional and/or sexual fantasies.

A complex and intricate array of biological, psychological, and social growths during puberty and adolescence lead to the emergence of the activation of sex energy <u>within</u> sexual desire. As stated in the introduction, sex *feels very, very good*. The question is, *why*? Let's examine what occurs when,

a) a man looks at a woman from a sexual point of view.
b) a woman looks at a man from a sexual point of view.
c) a man and woman look at each other from a sexual point of view.

When a man looks at a woman (or woman looks at a man) from a psycho-sexual viewpoint, there can be one of three possible mental responses: 1) *attraction response, 2) repulsion response, and 3) neutral response (non-attractive, non-repulsive response).* The **attraction response** (i.e. physical attraction) in men occurs when the senses are drawn toward the physical features of the woman. These physical features are: eye color, facial structure, breast size, overall physical shape, type of smile, type of perfume, dress, etc. The male mind becomes drawn toward female physical features, triggering the synthesis of semen. Semen exists in subtle form throughout the body and especially in the mind. This may seem like a strange statement. The term "**subtle semen**" has been created by the author to emphasize that sexual energy is generated out of neuropsychological processes. These processes exist within the subtle dimension (**sukshma sharara**) of one's being. Hence, "**subtle semen**" refers to energies within the brain/mind that ultimately are responsible for the synthesis and accumulation of sexual fluids in both men and women. Sexual fluids in themselves are part of the physical (gross) body and are the end result of extremely complex series of neurophysiological processes that are intrinsically connected to psycho-emotive functioning.

Of course, women do not produce semen, yet "**female ejaculation**" may exist in many women resulting from neuropsychological process that culminate in female orgasms. Suffice it to say, women can have prodigious sexual (orgasmic) energy flowing inside their bodies and minds based on levels of sexual arousal. For heterosexual men, orgasmic sexual energy takes the form of semen as their mind begins to think about the physical beauty of the female form. The man may even start to mentally fantasize (or, to put it another way, mentally masturbate) at the sight of an attractive woman. The more a man's mind engages in this process, it is to that extent the **subtle semen** flows to the genitals and creates the **gross semen** in the testicles. To reiterate, "**subtle semen**" refers to inherent neuropsychological energies existing in the brain and the spinal cord that are physiologically transformed into gross semen. This transformation of neurological energies into gross semen, via thought processes such as fantasy as well as stimulation of sexual organs, is responsible for the accumulation of semen in the testicles and the eventual climactic ejaculatory orgasm. This occurs, obviously, for reproduction. Yet, this process is not merely a non-experiential biological process. It is also a process that brings with it a very *personal and intimate* experience of **orgasmic pleasure**. From a "survival of the human species" perspective, human males are biologically, psychologically, and sexually programmed to "spread their seeds" (i.e. having **ejaculations**) for the survival of humanity. It is estimated that over 14 gallons of ejaculate is released from the male body in an average man's life. Semen is the end-product of this complex programming where food is transformed into sexual energy. The discharge of semen utilizes vast amounts of potent sexual energy for the purpose of procreation. Semen is a mixture of various fluids containing genetic material for reproduction that is ejaculated due to physical and psychological pressure. Physically, semen is created in the testicles, and it is discharged via stimulation of the penis. This stimulation, of course, can occur in many ways: oral sex, intercourse, masturbation, etc. The psychological process is much more complex and mysterious. The following questions highlight the mystery:

1) Why does the attraction response occur in the first place?
2) Once the attraction response takes place, what is the source of the experience of attraction?
3) What is happening in the mind that is causing a man to be "drawn toward" a woman and a woman to be "drawn toward" a man?

Let us examine the first question: "Why does the attraction response occur at all?" To answer this question, it is important to understand some truths about the nature of the mind. In general, the nature of the mind is such that it responds to the external world (including the opposite sex) with attraction, repulsion, or neutral responses. For example, when any man looks at any women, possible immediate reactions could be:

a) Wow!! She is hot!! (Sexual Attraction Response)
b) She is ok but not too attractive (Neutral Response)
c) She doesn't look that great… (Negative Response)
d) I could never be with her…. (Repulsive Response)

Such instant reactions occur within the mind of most men simply based on physical structure and looks. (A similar response occurs in women when they see a man.) The psychological mystery is simply, *why does this happen at all?* According to many spiritual traditions, the answer can be found only when an individual becomes a student of his/her own mind (and a student of desires embedded within the mind) by performing spiritual practices such as meditation, introspection, self-observation, self-reflection, etc. so that the *answer* to this question is found *intuitively.* Many spiritual traditions state that once an individual realizes that the source of the attraction is in the mind and it is the *mind itself* that is causing the individual to be drawn, "entrapped," and "snared" in the charms of the woman (or man), then a deeper realization occurs about the nature of this attraction. This deeper realization then, as it is claimed by many spiritualists, will allow the individual to transcend sexual desires and enter into a "trans-desire state" where deep bondage of sexual desire is shattered.

Each person is intimately familiar with his/her own sexuality and pleasure experienced in sexual stimulation. The pursuit of sexual pleasure is instinctually innate and highly mysterious. The mystery of sex unfolds in exploring several basic questions that humans have grappled with throughout history. These questions are:

a) Why does sex feel good? Why is there experience of pleasure?
b) Where is the origin of the experience of sexual pleasure?
c) What triggers sexual process to start (i.e. getting turned on) within an individual?
d) Why does human procreation necessarily involve the experience of orgasmic pleasures? What possible reasons exist as to why orgasmic pleasure coincides with the act of procreation?
e) Do animals feel pleasure in their sex act?
f) Is the residing place of sexual desire in the brain or the mind? Is the mind something different from the brain, and do humans have free will regarding their sexuality?
g) What happens if an individual completely suppresses sexual impulses? Does it cause psychological, emotional, and/or physical problems?
h) What happens if individuals keep little or no boundaries on sexual activity? Will this lead to complete chaos in society and cause massive familial, psychological, economic, and spiritual problems for individuals?
i) Is there a Supreme Being (God or Super Soul) that has placed sexual desire within each human being for the purpose of reproduction? If so, why do major world religions place certain restrictions on sexual activity?
j) Is there a way to unlock nearly endless sexual (orgasmic) pleasure within oneself by specific yogic or meditation practices?

All these questions have been contemplated and debated for thousands of years, having major implications within multiple dimensions of one's life. Before we can dive into these questions, it is prudent to begin our exploration by first learning about the sexual response cycle in the next chapter. Clear understanding of the sexual response cycle is at the heart of intrinsically unfolding hidden mysteries of **sex energy** and **orgasmic ecstasy**.

To becomes aware of one's own mental processes is the greatest blessing one can give to oneself. There is nothing more precious than energy that exists in one's own mind and body. The most potent form of energy is one's own sex energy. It can be used constructively or destructively. The choice is ours.

-- Sachin J. Karnik

Attraction and repulsion are polarities of the mind. Energy moves in this polarity where it gets concentrated and fragmented, and its quality changes significantly, thereby causing multiple effects throughout one's biological, psychological, and sociological systems.

-- Sachin J. Karnik

CHAPTER 2

OVERVIEW OF SEXUAL RESPONSE

SEXUAL RESPONSE CYCLE

Understanding human sexuality necessitates examining what is known as the **"sexual response cycle."** This cycle is technically defined as:

"A pattern of physiologic events occurring during sexual arousal and intercourse. In both men and women, these events may be identified as occurring in a sequence of four stages: excitement, plateau, orgasm, and resolution. The basic pattern of these stages is similar in both sexes, regardless of the specific sexual stimulus.[2]" (see Figure 1)

FIGURE 1
HUMAN SEXUAL RESPONSE CYCLE

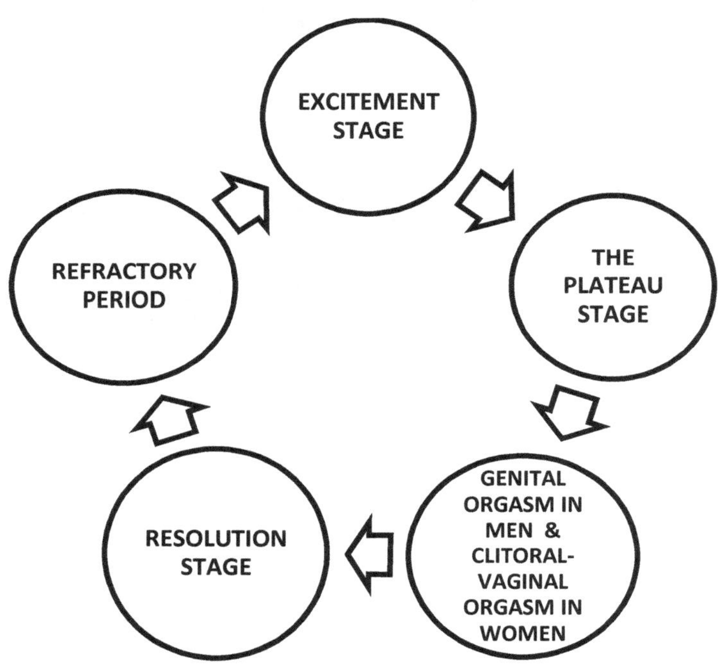

The 5 phases of the sexual response cycle are shown above, as illustrated by Masters and Johnson. (The purpose of pre-orgasmic stimulation (for men) is to remain in the plateau state and pull small pieces of orgasmic currents from the next state without entering into a "genital orgasm" that results in a "negative relaxation" (i.e. the resolution state). So, the refractory period, in the usual sense, is avoided. This is discussed in chapter 7 of this book.)

The term "**human sexual response cycle**" was coined by William H. Masters and Virginia E. Johnson in their 1966 book *Human Sexual Response*. These researchers conducted extensive observational studies to unravel the intricacies of human sexual response. From the definition of the cycle as shown above, we can clearly see a "pattern of physiologic events" taking place. *Physiologic events* refer to intricate physiological and neurological processes taking place from the start of the cycle to the end of the cycle. There are changes in blood pressure, heart rate, breathing (shallowness and rapidity of breath), and of course, changes in both male and female sex organs.

In the above definition, the term **"sexual arousal"** refers to **sexual desire** being produced, stimulated, and awakened due to anticipating sexual activity or during sexual activity. Sexual arousal can become active due to a variety of stimuli that cause an erotic response. In conventional terms, this is known as being "turned on." Stimuli can be mental, physical, or both that may lead to sexual arousal which in turn may lead to **orgasm** if increased stimulation occurs. No doubt there are many changes within a person that are subtle in nature (i.e., movement of thoughts in one direction) and changes that are more pronounced physically (i.e., blood pressure and heart rate). Of course, sexual arousal does not always lead people to act upon their arousal. They may merely want to remain in the arousal state for some time, and then return to a pre-arousal state. Once aroused, if there is sufficient stimulation then an orgasm would most likely occur. An understanding of the sexual response cycle is foundational to clearly exploring major ideas presented in chapters 3-9. Therefore, the author recommends spending some time in clearly understanding each state of the sexual response cycle.

EXCITEMENT STAGE

A thought or a memory of a sexual encounter or the sight of a sexually appealing person can be enough to start sexual excitement within oneself. This excitement is one's *personal experience*. Take a moment and try to remember the feeling of becoming sexually excited. This process is highly personal and based on the subjective nature of one's inner desires. Once the process begins, there are physiological changes in one's sexual organs and other parts of the body. The excitement preceding sexual climax has its origin in the anticipation of at least the following three things: a) the experience of orgasmic pleasure, b) fulfillment of built up sexual pressure requiring release, and c) satisfaction of deep-seated sexual cravings. Of course, there are certainly many other reasons for the awakening of sexual excitement where the three reasons just mentioned are largely predominant in most people. Also, in examining male-female relationships, an enormous amount of time, energy, money, and thought goes into planning for a sexual encounter. All this preparation itself is exciting, and it precedes what is known as the "excitement stage" in the sexual response cycle.

The **excitement stage** is defined as follows:

"In the excitement stage, the body prepares for sexual activity by tensing muscles and increasing heart rate and blood pressure. In the male, blood flows into the penis, causing it to become erect; in the female, the vaginal walls become moist, the inner part of the vagina becomes wider, and the clitoris enlarges.[3]"

The excitement stage (phase) is also known as the "arousal phase or the initial excitement phase" as it is the first stage of the human sexual response cycle. As discussed earlier, this arousal or excitement is a direct result of diverse types of physical and/or mental stimuli that are erotic in nature. These can include petting, kissing, and/or viewing erotic images that lead to sexual excitement. In this excitement state, the physical body and the mind are preparing for what is known as "**coitus or sexual intercourse**" that occurs in the next phase known as the "plateau phase."[4]

PLATEAU STAGE

As excitement builds up, there is also an increase in the amount of pleasure experienced as the body/mind prepare to enter into what is known as the "**point-of-no-return**" in men. (See Figure 3) The **point-of-no-return** is a climax point where orgasm and ejaculation occur simultaneously in men. Hence, the excitement state leads to the plateau stage which then leads to the **orgasmic stage**. The **plateau stage** is an extension of the excitement stage and is defined as follows:

"In the plateau stage, breathing becomes more rapid and the muscles continue to tense; the glans at the head of the penis swells and the testes enlarge in the male; in the female, the outer vagina contracts and the clitoris retracts.[5]"

Clearly, there are significant changes in breathing rate, muscle tension, penis size, and testicle size in men. All these changes in men occur to ensure semen insertion into the woman's vagina for reproduction. These changes are simultaneously accompanied by intimate experiences of increasing pleasure that culminate into highly concentrated sexual climax. In men, this climax provides a potent orgasmic experience with semen discharge. In women, there are changes in the outer vagina and the clitoris with increasing pre-orgasmic pleasure.

Concentration of sex energy occurs during the excitement stage. Revitalization of this energy occurs when one is directly in touch with the onset of the concentration process. Enhancing cognizance and attentiveness of sex energy churning within oneself is a form of meditation.
-- Sachin J. Karnik

ORGASMIC STAGE
(GENITAL ORGASM IN MEN AND CLITORAL-VAGINAL ORGASM IN WOMEN)

As stimulation continues and sexual excitation increases, the entire process culminates into an "**orgasm**." In men, orgasm and ejaculation occur simultaneously, yet they are different processes. This simultaneous occurrence is due to ensuring the survival of the human species. Potent pleasure is experienced in an ejaculatory orgasm, specifically, to ensure that semen is discharged. In women, there may or may not be discharge of sexual fluids, yet the orgasmic experience is quite similar. **Orgasm**, for both men and women can be defined as follows:

"At orgasm, neuromuscular tension built up in the preceding stages is released in a few seconds. In the woman, the vagina begins a series of regular contractions; in the man, the penis also contracts rhythmically to expel the sperm and semen (ejaculation).[6]"

This straightforward definition clearly highlights the existence of "neuromuscular tension" during orgasm. This tension exists due to the concentration of sex energies demanding release. A very specific type of mental focus is required for an orgasm to occur. This focus creates neuromuscular tension and interestingly, the same focus also releases this tension. The author encourages the reader to see for oneself the emergence and enhancement of this special type of mental focus and the movement of energy within it. The mind finds a deepening oneness with one's partner (actual or imagined) as sexual stimulation increases and approaches orgasm (sexual climax).

Orgasm, then, can be thought of as any or all the following:

1) Orgasm can be one brief moment of extreme pleasure experienced just after the building of excitement and tension, *just before* the deep post-orgasmic relaxation, and *just before* the psychological release of sex energy.

2) Orgasms create physical changes in heart rate, blood pressure, skin color, muscle contractions, etc. These physical changes are part of the usual orgasmic experience.

3) In men, ejaculation of semen is usually accompanied by a genital orgasm.

4) Orgasm can be thought of as an emotional or even as a spiritual experience according to some spiritual traditions of the world.

5) Orgasms undoubtedly have universal appeal where substantial time, effort, money, and energy are expended on trying to experience pleasure inherent within orgasmic experiences. Hence, the term, "**orgasmic pleasure**" refers to the intense sexual pleasure that is part of the orgasmic phase. There are certainly many types of pleasure. Orgasmic experiences are part of

the overall experience of sex pleasure. Deep psychological demands exist for the repetition and enhancement of orgasmic pleasures.

6) Orgasm can be understood in a medical or physiological sense based on understanding processes within the body. As stated before, there are changes in body temperature, heart rate, skin flush, changes in hormones, changes in sensitivity of the sexual organs, muscle contractions, etc. There are still no universally accepted measurements for orgasms, nevertheless, all these changes have been used by scientists to "prove" that an orgasm has occurred. Of course, this mere physiological definition would mean that if one's body changes based on certain criteria, then an individual has had an orgasm. One can certainly see the limitations of this definition in that it does not account for personal experience, personal sensation, and personal pleasure that is imbedded with an orgasm. The physiological changes, of course, do occur and must be considered as valid for an orgasm, yet it may be possible to have the same physiological changes without the person experiencing orgasm or orgasmic pleasure.[7]

7) Orgasm can also be understood from a psychological perspective, and it could be conceptualized based on an individual's subjective experiences of satisfaction, release of psychic pressure/tension, release of emotional tensions, etc. with deep satisfaction of desires. It is interesting to note that Sigmund Freud identified two distinct types of orgasms in women: vaginal orgasms and clitoral orgasms. Freud considered vaginal orgasms to be a sign of good psychological and emotional health; whereas, he considered mere clitoral orgasms to be a sign that proper psychosocial development had not occurred or had been hindered. Most psychological researchers and mental health professionals have abandoned Freud's view and state that a person can be said to have a healthy orgasm based on self-report and subjective experience.[8]

RESOLUTION STAGE

Having explored the orgasmic stage along some possible characteristics of orgasms, the next phase of the sexual response cycle is known as the "**resolution stage**" of the sexual response cycle. The resolution phase is conceptualized as follows:

"The succeeding **resolution stage** brings a gradual return to the resting state that may take several hours. In the male, the penis shrinks back to its normal size; in the female, the vagina and other genital structures also return to their pre-excitement condition.[9]"

The resolution phase occurs after peak experience of an orgasm when ejaculation (in men) has occurred and after multiple orgasms have occurred in women. Emphasis should be placed on the fact that the resolution phase in women will vary, based on a variety of factors such as hormonal balance, level of desire, type of satisfaction experienced, and other factors that can be self-perceived. The returning of the vagina and other genital structures in women back to resting state are the outward manifestations of having reached sexual peaks where the desire to again reach orgasmic peaks is diminished significantly or absent. Hence, this is a possible resolution state in women.

REFRACTORY PERIOD

As the resolution stage comes to an end, a "**refractory period**" occurs primarily in men. This refractory period is conceptualized as follows:

"The resolution stage in men contains a **refractory period** of several minutes to a few hours, during which the man is incapable of further sexual arousal. Women have no such refractory period and can quickly become aroused again from any point in the resolution stage.[10]"

A refractory period in women is considerably different in men compared to women, such that women can become sexually aroused again while being in the resolution stage. This is a noteworthy difference because men enter the refractory period after having an ejaculation that is accompanied simultaneously by a peak orgasm. The peak experience of orgasm with ejaculation in men results in men entering the refractory period due to having large amounts of neuro-physiological and psychological energies concentrated into a highly focused process, so that semen is discharged from the male penis with a tremendous sense of satisfaction of deep-seated sexual desire. It can be stated that the refractory period is a state of mind where desire for further sexual activity is not present due to a deep sense of **satiation**. Satiation is the full satisfaction of an appetite or desire; and at times, the word "satiation" can also be used to specify that satisfaction is taken to an excess, yet this is a secondary meaning of the word. The sexual response cycle, particularly in men, intends to discharge semen, resulting in a state of satiation of sexual desires/impulses, and possibly leading to a profound sense of tension relief and satisfaction. Hence, the state of satisfaction is a temporary state of desirelessness. Along with this state of desirelessness, there is also a significant usage of energy that needs to be replenished by consuming diverse types of food. Of course, the daily consumption of food and the *energy locked up in food* is used for a multitude of physiological and psychological processes. The experience of ejaculatory orgasm utilizes significant amounts of energy. This energy utilization is due to a deep-rooted command structures in the brain that are responsible for dispelling semen for the purpose of reproduction. Such deep-rooted processes exist for the survival of the human species.

One crucial point worth noting is that the resolution phase in some women may reach a similar state of satiation after prolonged multiple orgasms have occurred. It is also possible that some women may experience such a state of satiation from just one or a few orgasms. The point made in the definition above is simply that *most* (not all) women can become aroused from any point in the resolution state.

It is important to note that the sexual response cycle within each person is mostly identical irrespective of **sexual orientation**, **LBGTQ** identification, and/or diverse means of achieving arousal (i.e. masturbation, view of pornographic materials, multiple partners, etc.) The cycle may function differently based on physical health conditions and emotional states, yet the stages of the cycle occur with consistency.

HEDONIC SET POINT – DESIRE – PLEASURE – AROUSAL – ORGASM – REFRACTION

An additional way of understanding sexual response is as follows:

1) Wanting → Liking → Learning
2) Expectation → Consummation → Satiety
3) Desire → Arousal → Plateau → Orgasm → Refraction

A **hedonic set point** exists when each person. As sexual desire increases, pleasure also increases leading to the hedonic set point. This is a point where sexual desire culminates into the *onset* of sexual pleasure. This set point is modified and changed based on types of stimulation and subjective experiences of pleasure. The diagram below illustrates that increase in sexual desire (via internal and/or external triggers) takes the mind toward the hedonic set point. "Wanting" and "expectation" are prominent in this stage.

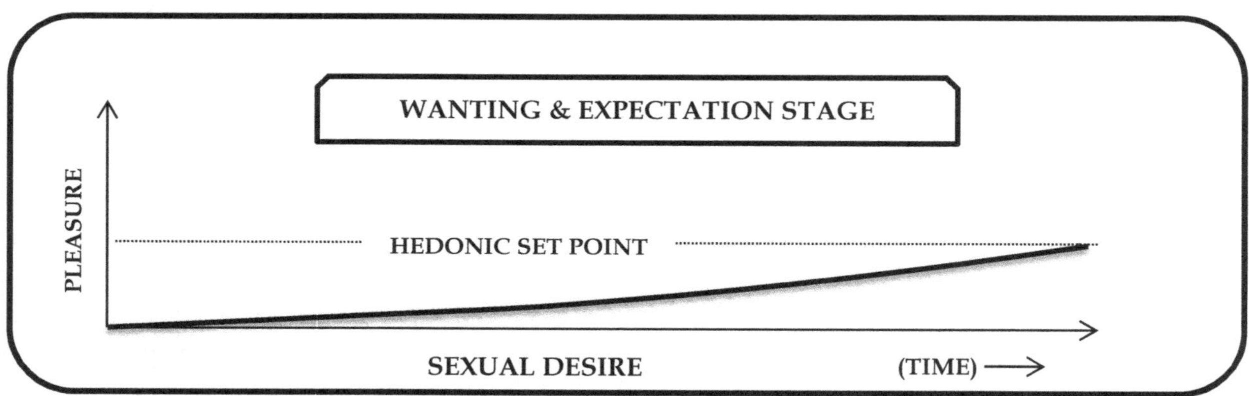

The words "sexual pleasure" and "sexual desire" are linguistic representations of internal phenomena that are beyond language. Language utterly pales compared to direct experience. -- Sachin J. Karnik

The diagram below illustrates the "wanting and liking" stage that exists after the hedonic set point is reached. This is a stage of arousal where pleasure is substantially increased.

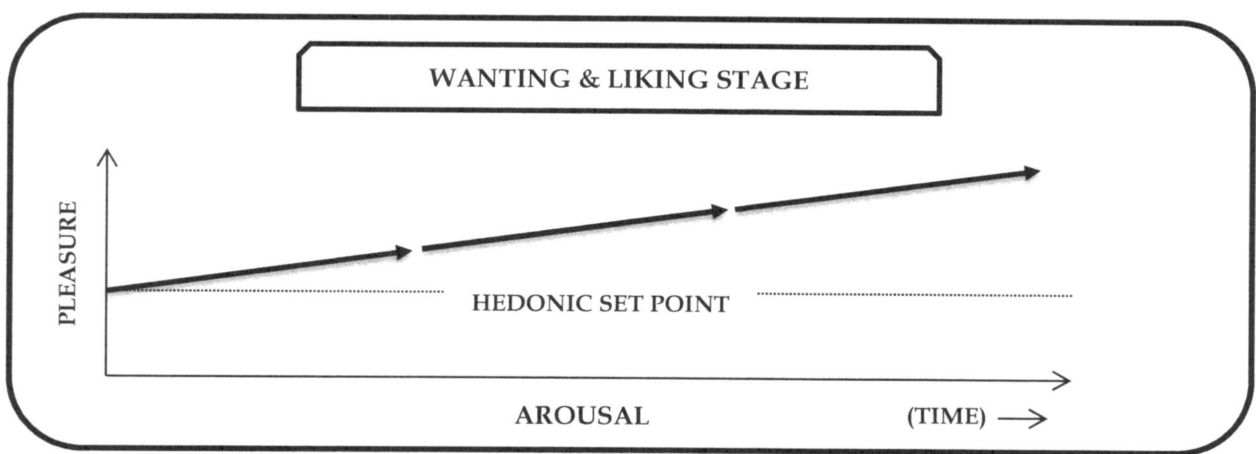

The diagram below illustrates the "liking and consummation state" where one is aroused and can remain in a state of arousal. This is the plateau stage where desire for peak orgasm gets gradually stronger.

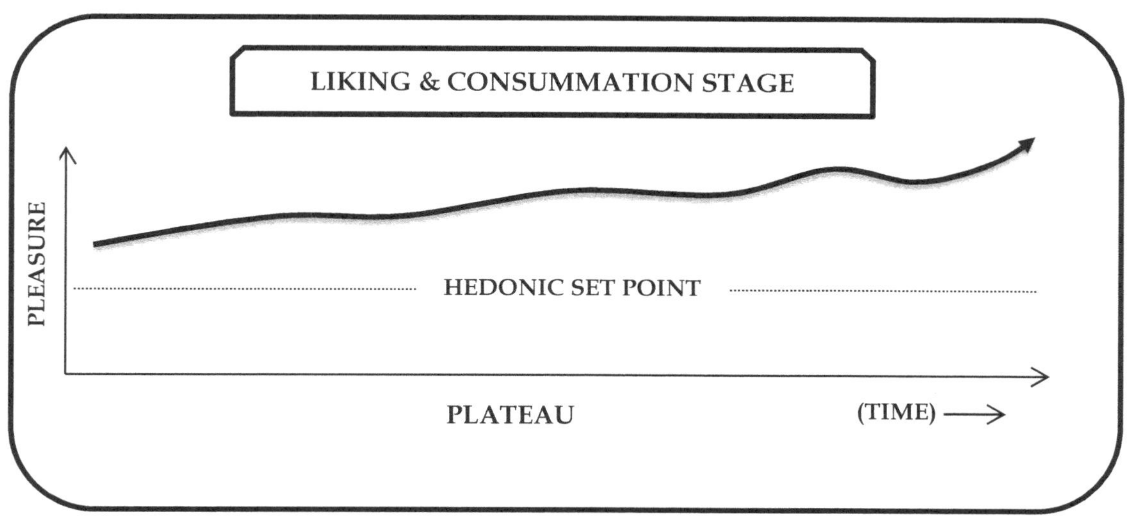

Pure love has no friction. It is one's own essential nature existing within the substratum of reality itself. Is there friction in the plateau stage? -- Sachin J. Karnik

The diagram below illustrates the orgasmic stage where "peak liking and peak consummation" occur. Peak experience occurs much beyond the hedonic set point. **Orgasm** occurs at this peak.

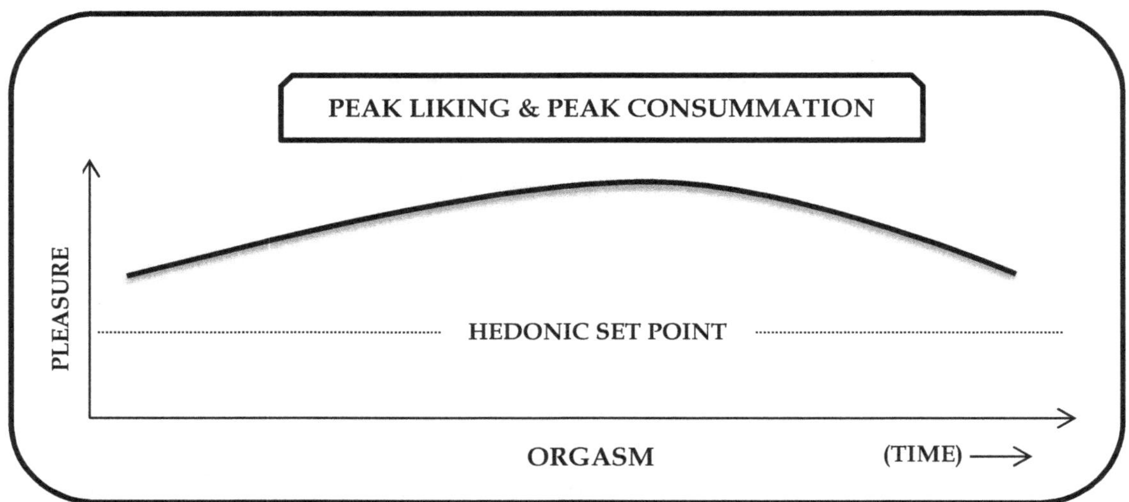

The diagram below illustrates the refractory period where "learning and satiety" occur. "Learning" refers to remembering the steps that are required to reach orgasm. This is necessary for the sexual response cycle to restart after a temporary refractory period. "Satiety" refers to a state of satisfaction where no further desire for orgasm is present. In men, this occurs in an ejaculatory orgasm; and in women this occurs after multiple orgasms, based on hormonal levels and overall level of psychological non-disturbance.

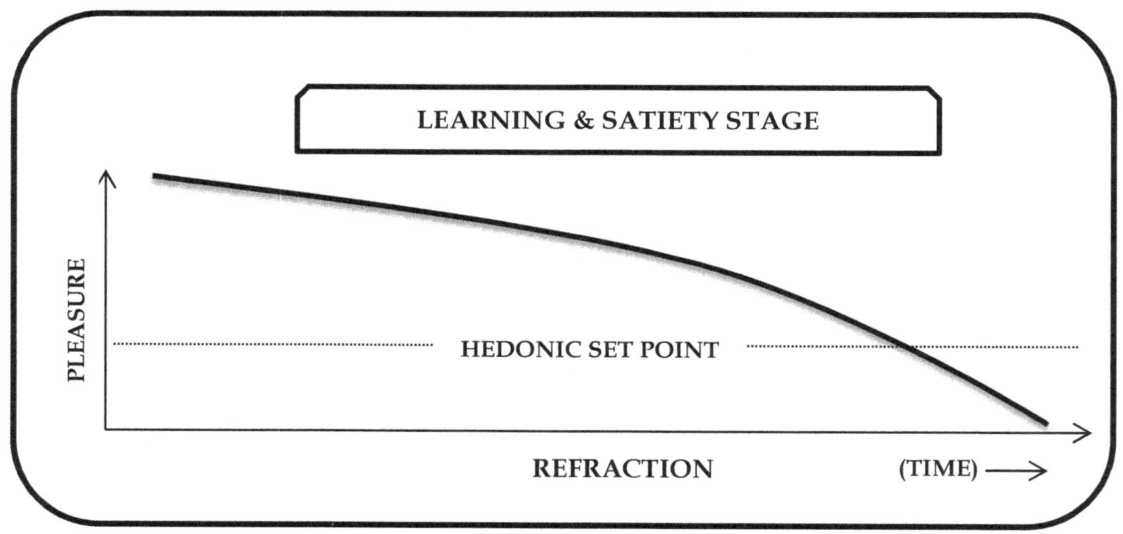

CHAPTER 3

EJACULATORY ORGASMS, POINT-OF-NO-RETURN, & MEDITATIVE SEXUAL PRACTICES

> ***The mind is a great mystery. Positive energy within one's mind can take one to great heights. Negativity degrades this energy and imprisons the mind where the mind torments itself and others.***
>
> ***Sachin J. Karnik***

THE SEX-ORGASM-CELIBACY (BRAHMACHARYA) CONTINUUM IN MEN

Having examined the sexual response cycle, let's continue further by examining "**The Sex-Orgasm-Celibacy Continuum.**" Figure 2, shown below, depicts this continuum in men. (Please see the next section for women).

FIGURE 2

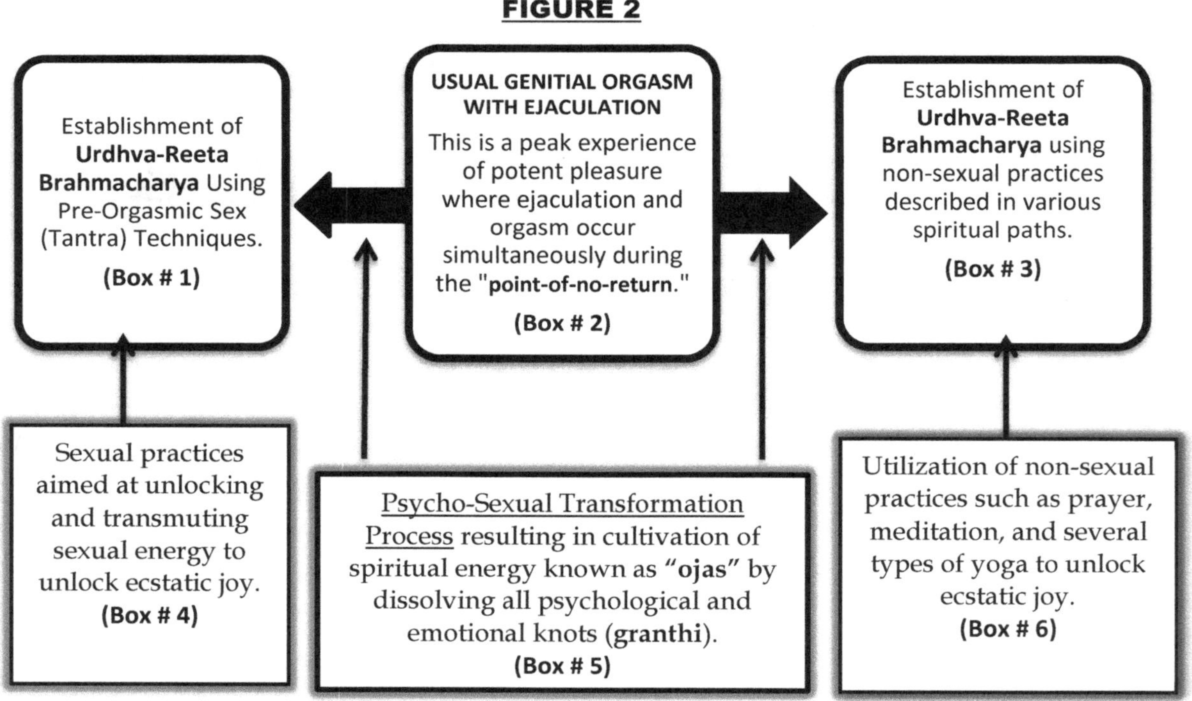

For Men:

At first glance, the diagram above has three words (**Urdhva-Reeta Brahmacharaya)** that may be totally unfamiliar to you. Before examining the meaning of these words, let us begin by examining box # 2. In this box is written, "usual genital orgasm with ejaculation" that primarily refers to male ejaculatory orgasm. Most men are in box # 2 where their sexual activity occurs according to processes described in the sexual response cycle with peak experiences of ejaculatory orgasm. (Note: women generally can have peak experiences of orgasms without significant reduction in sexual desire. The reduction or temporary extinction of desire is usually experienced by men during the refractory period.) Also within box # 2 there is a statement about the "**point-of-no-return**." (Please see Figure 3 as shown below.)

FIGURE 3 – POINT-OF-NO-RETURN

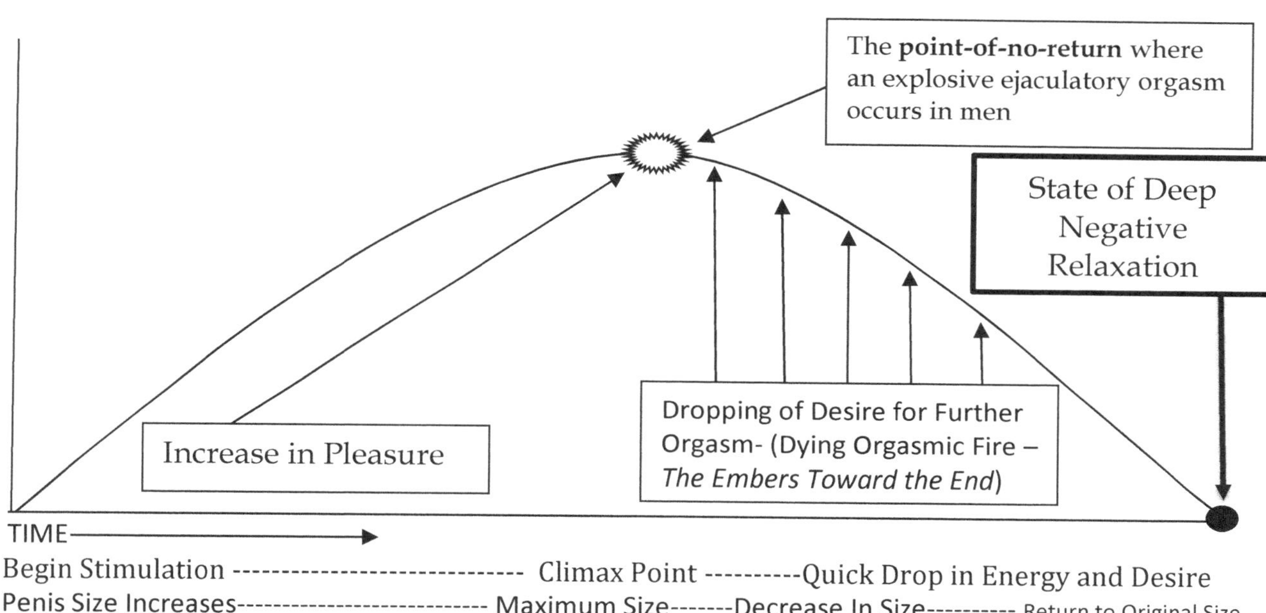

The **point-of-no-return** specifically applies to men. It is a mental/neurological trigger where **orgasmic inevitability** and **ejaculatory inevitability** have taken place, and it is nearly impossible to prevent a peak orgasm with ejaculation. It is important to be very clear that men have a concentrated peak experience in the sexual response cycle. After the peak experience, there emerges naturally, a **refractory period** that come with a subjective sense of negative relaxation. This **negative relaxation** is due to the release of sexual pressure, release of neuropsychological and physiological energy, and of course, semen discharge for the purpose of **procreation**. As stated before, women also have a refractory period, yet they can enter into the orgasmic phase rather quickly without a significant loss of energy and desire that usually occurs in most men in the refractory period. To be clear, the writer is not stating in any way that there is anything wrong with the usual sexual response cycle, or that it is unnatural or harmful in any way. To some extent, each person is familiar with his/her own sexual response cycle. Increased awareness of one's own sexual responses allows for progress to be made in unlocking one's sexual potential.

In further examining box # 2, we can see that males will enter the **point-of-no-return** followed by a significant reduction in the intensity of desire along with release of sexual tension. There can also exist a deep state of relaxation and an *exquisite* feeling of mental silence, accompanied by deep satisfaction that comes with the ejaculatory orgasm. Of course, this is completely natural. The state of deep psychological silence that is usually experienced after an ejaculatory orgasm is a temporary state where the activity of sexual desire is temporarily non-functional or minimally functional, for most men. Again, the extent of the refractory period varies among men, ranging from minutes to days before sexual desire increases substantially.

In examining boxes 1 and 3, the term, "***urdhva-reeta brahmacharya***" is written. This is a **Sanskrit** term that refers to a state of total transformation of sexual desire and sexual energy in men. (This state is also possible for women and is discussed in the next section.) Each of these three words can be understood as follows:

Urdhva = up
Reetas = sexual essences and energies
Brahmacharya = a state of functioning of the entire psycho-sexual system where total sublimation, transformation, **transmutation**, and purification of sexual desires, pleasures, and energies occur with the possibility of opening a doorway into the spiritual dimension that exists beyond limited thought and emotion.

These three words combined refer to a state of total conservation of sexual energies with the ultimate aim of spiritual transformation. This conservation can be accomplished by two diametrically opposite paths that have the same goal of using sex energy for greater internal awakening. Box # 1 refers to the "left-handed path" where sexual practices are used to conserve and transmute energies. These sexual practices are part of the Eastern spiritual tradition known as **tantra** and also part of the **Taoist** tradition. The word "**tantra**" refers to integration and the "weaving together" of fragmented psychological energies using pleasure itself to move beyond limited pleasure into a state of **orgasmic ecstasy**. The connections between Box 1 and Box 2 are shown below (Figure 4) as a transformative process moving from stage 1 to stage 7:

There is a vast difference between "change" and "transformation." Change is like a caterpillar moving from one point to another. Transformation is the caterpillar getting stabilized in one place, spinning a cocoon around itself, and becoming a butterfly. The butterfly does not become a caterpillar again. Orgasm can transform into ecstasy and ecstasy can transform into undiluted joy.

-- Sachin J. Karnik

FIGURE 4
(MEDITATIVE SEXUAL PRACTICES FOR MEN)

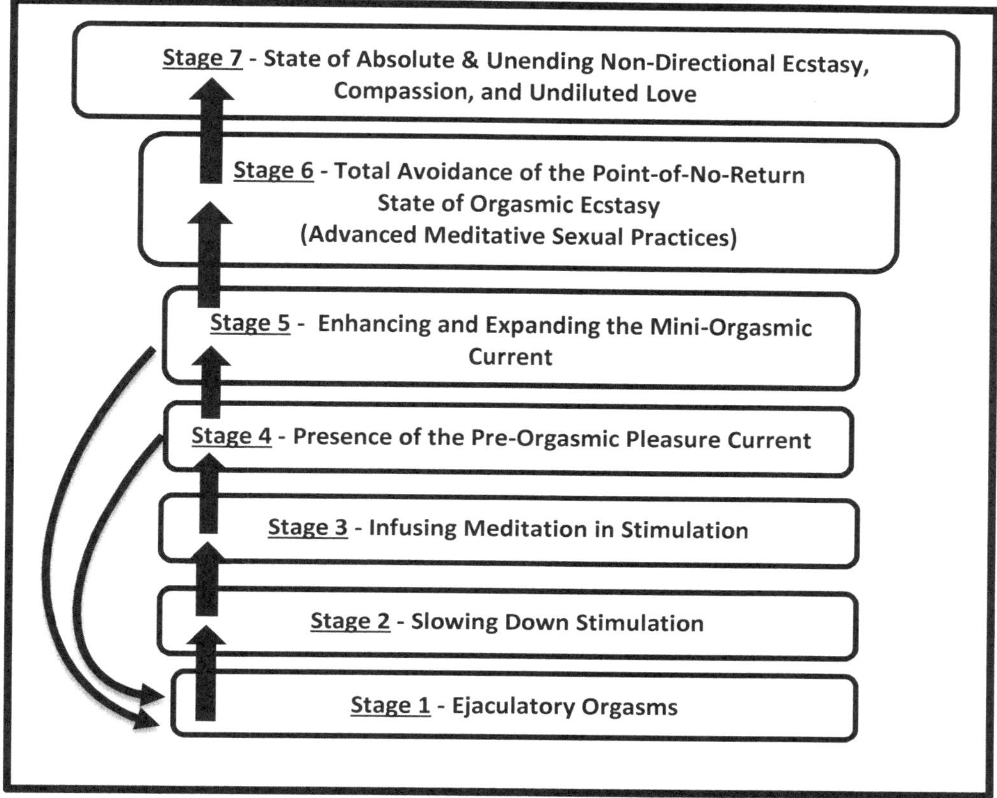

This diagram shows a gradual transition from mere ejaculatory orgasms to a state of **orgasmic ecstasy**, which has the potential of leading to a state of absolute love as indicated in box # 7 above. The specifics of this practice are covered in Chapter 7. Suffice it to say, the body and mind become charged with orgasmic energy by remaining in a pre-orgasmic state for extended periods of time. This allows for **valley orgasms** to occur naturally along with simultaneous cultivation of sexual essences. This cultivation of sexual essences, while experiencing valley orgasms (or mini-orgasms), is possible in the male body. Prevention of the refractory period via slow and meditative stimulation with awareness of the movements of orgasmic currents, provides for cultivation and rejuvenation of sexual desire. Most men are unaware of this possibility. Various practices described in Chapter 7 show step-by-step methods in becoming proficiently established in pre-orgasmic stimulation with cultivation of sexual essences. The process of transforming male semen by allowing the male body to reabsorb the semen is the essence of perfect meditative (tantric) lovemaking where orgasmic experiences become wider while sexual essences are cultivated and transmuted. Consequently, the word "**brahmacharya**" refers to perfection in retaining what is known as **bindu**. **Bindu** is the **Sanskrit** word for all the following:

1) Male semen or the "**ejaculate**."
2) The neuropsychological energy in the brain and the spinal cord responsible for orgasmic and ejaculatory experiences in men.
3) The portion of energy utilized by the body in creating the semen and eventually ejaculating it.

Given these three ways **bindu** is described, understanding the term "**tantric yoga**" is necessary. This term refers to practices of **yoga** (i.e. union or connection) and **tantra** (i.e. weaving together) that are aimed at perfecting the process of retaining the **bindu**. The **tantric yogi** (i.e. person who mixes meditation and pleasure) is an individual who is extremely careful not to lose his **semen (i.e. bindu)** at any cost and sees the importance of totally sublimating semen (**bindu**). Sex energy conservation (i.e. **Brahmacharya**), in the tantric mode, is where sex energy is retained and recirculated. This retention and recirculation increases neuropsychological energy and increases storage of this energy. Climactic and explosive male ejaculatory orgasm is a deep release of this energy. It is theorized that those who practice this type of sexual continence while enjoying orgasmic pleasures may have enhanced physical and mental strength, increased splendor, increased endurance, and greater vitality. These are manifestations of such heightened strength. Of course, this type of complete sex energy sublimation in men is extremely rare. Some spiritual practitioners aim to conserve and sublimate their entire sexual energy for the purpose of spiritual transformation.

Sex, by itself, has the primary purpose of reproduction and these practices of sex sublimation may not be your goal as such. Even then, the practices shown later on in this book can be utilized to make some movement upwards from stage 1 to state 4 where the presence of the **mini-orgasmic pleasure current** eventually occurs. If one climbs up to stage 4 and is totally satisfied with recirculating sexual energies while allowing for mini-orgasmic pleasure currents to arise for a certain period of time and then eventually decides to have a powerful ejaculatory orgasm, then that can be very gratifying. Progressing up to stage 4 is an indication of increased progress in enhancing sexual pleasures. If one is so inclined, one can go further to expand mini-orgasmic pleasure currents flowing through the entire body. When one enters stage 5, more potent and powerful mini-orgasmic pleasure currents occur that can be repeatedly experienced. At this level of mastery of orgasmic waves, levels of orgasmic pleasure can be up to 95% of ejaculatory orgasm! (This statement is made based on many personal accounts of people adept at meditative sex. There has not been enough research performed to determine a percentage number due to the relatively few people who are aiming to reach stage 5.)

If one can remain in stage 5 without any discharge (or very minimal discharge) of semen, then sex energy is going through **transmutation/transformation**. In this state, repeated experiences of orgasmic pleasure continue as unblocking of psychological knots (**granthi**) occurs. This unlocking and unblocking of major psychological/emotional knots (blocks) leads to stage 6 where **orgasmic ecstasy** will arise and begin to overflow in all directions in one's life as stage 7 is approached. In stage 7, there can be an abiding state of non-directional ecstasy. In this ecstasy, opening of undiluted love and compassion occurs. An ejaculatory orgasm is merely a fragment of this pure state of love. In other words, an enlightened **tantric yogi** (i.e. one who has masterfully mixed meditation with pleasure) is one who is living in a state of undiluted and non-fragmentary love. This is what is meant by non-direction love. Generally, our "love" is directional, in the sense that we "love" someone or a few people, yet do not have the same feeling for others. This is, of course, natural, and there is no criticism of it. Nonetheless, for those who are aiming to enter into an evolved state of emotion where emotion transforms from revolving within a boundary to evolving into a state where limited psychological boundaries fall off, deep appreciation of the importance and glory of non-directional flow of love is obligatory.

Consider the following: directional movement of sex energy is pleasure; non-directional flow of sex energy is beyond pleasure and is a state of sublimated pleasure or refined pleasure. *Remember, all of this is a matter of personal experience and exploration*. If one truly progresses beyond stage 4, then, in the opinion of the writer, one enters into the **Sex Knot (Granthi) Dissolution Cycle in Men** (See Figure 5 below).

(NOTE: The dissolution of the sex knot is also possible in women. In the opinion of the author, this transformative dissolution of the sex knot occurs naturally as progress occurs in meditative sexuality. This progress is shown in Figure 6.)

Immense energy is funneled and concentrated into the sex knot, creating orgasmic experiences. The dissolving of the sex knot releases unimaginable energy in which natural ecstasy abides constantly. This is not suppression of sex desire. It is deep transformation of it.

-- Sachin J. Karnik

FIGURE 5
THE SEX KNOT *(GRANTHI)* DISSOLUTION CYCLE IN MEN
(Each Circle Is Explained by Number Below)

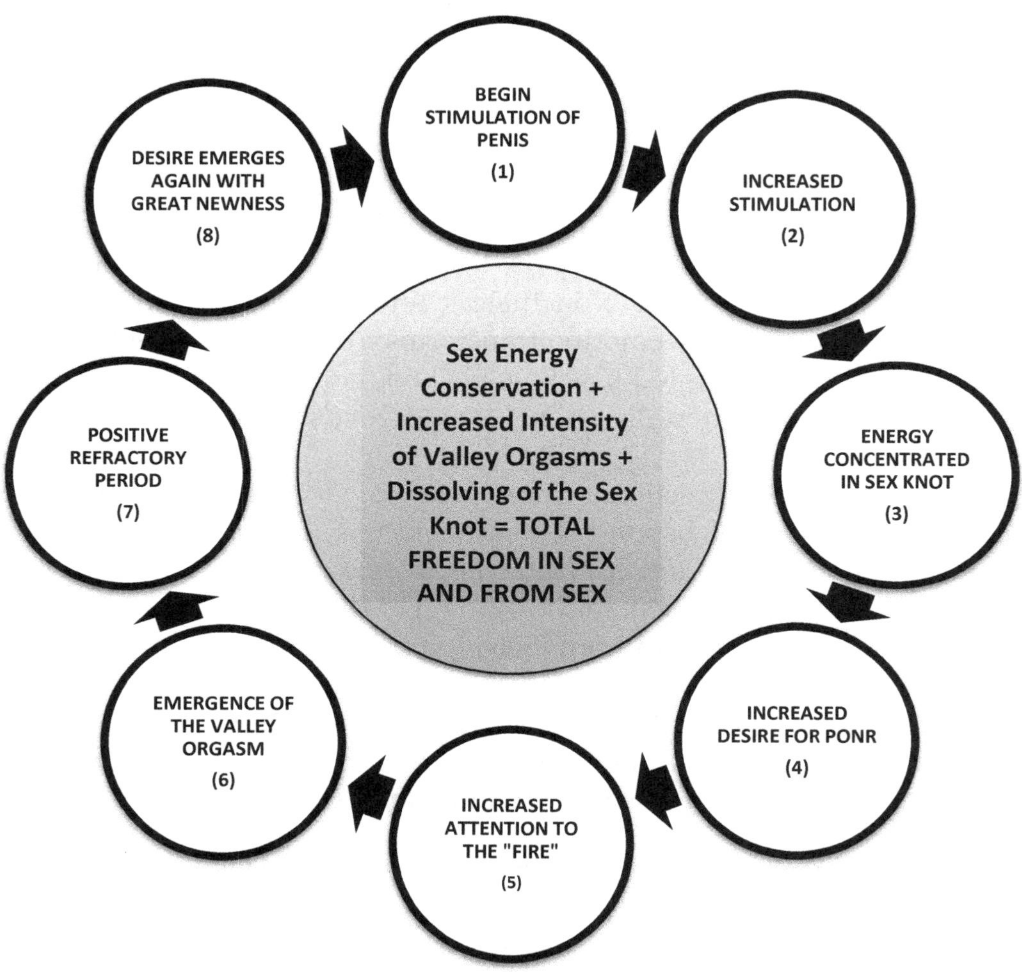

1) <u>*Penis Stimulation*</u>: This has to be done carefully with a great deal of meditative awareness of the movement of energy and pleasure within the body.
2) <u>*Increased Stimulation*</u>: With increased stimulation comes greater pleasure and requires greater mastery in approaching the **point-of-no return** and keeping away from it, allowing for **valley orgasms** to flower naturally.
3) <u>***The Sex Knot***</u>: Increase in focus of orgasmic energy currents due to movement of energy through the sex knot. This sex knot is known as **Hridaya Granthi** in scriptures from India. There is considered to be a major intra-psychic block that concentrates energy and prevents sex energy transmutation.
4) <u>*Increased Desire to Reach the Point-Of-No-Return*</u>: This desire exists for the purpose of procreation. The male mind is immersed in excitation aimed at reaching the climax point where ejaculation and orgasm occur together.
5) <u>*The "Fire" in the Beginning*</u>: By keeping attention to the "fire in the beginning" (i.e. mini-orgasmic currents), the **point-of-no-return** is intelligently avoided. As orgasmic energy gets funneled in the knot, the attention to mini-orgasmic currents causes the energy to move out of the knot and not remain concentrated.

6) *Emergence of Valley Orgasm*: Mini-orgasmic currents begin to move throughout the body. As the cycle is repeated over and over again, the **point-of-no-return** is avoided and psychic energy (mental energy) is not discharged. The sex knot begins to dissolve as whole-body orgasms occur without ejaculation. These orgasmic currents create **valley orgasms** that have anywhere from 50% to 95% of pleasure of a full ejaculatory orgasm. These smaller orgasms intensify every time they are repeated and can potentially reoccur for extended periods of time. Eventually, a break must be taken to relax, yet **positive relaxation** is required, and one may start the cycle anytime due to the fact that the potency of desire remains active.
7) *Positive Refractory Period*: There is a positive refractory period where energy is conserved, transformed, and male sexual fluids are re-absorbed into the body. This reabsorption is the core process of **brahmacharya** where sexual essences are transmuted into **ojas** energy.
8) *Desire Emerges with Great Newness:* The "newness" of desire is experienced due to avoiding negative refraction.

NOTE: Sex Energy Conservation + Increased Intensity of Valley Orgasms + Dissolving of the Sex Knot = FREEDOM

The term "**Sex Knot**" is known as "**hridaya granthi**" in ancient Hindu scriptures and it is translated as the "knot of the heart." The "**sex knot**" refers to human beings remaining "stuck in limited sexuality" (i.e. box 2 in the Sex-Orgasm-Celibacy Continuum"). There are many energy knots or blocks within one's personality structure. These energy knots are intersection points where energy and consciousness intermingle and manifest in a variety of ways. The total unraveling of these energy knots is the end result of moving successfully through the sex knot dissolution cycle. There is a central pathway within each person, existing in subtle dimensions, known as the **Sushumna-Nadi,** which is considered to be a central spiritual nerve that has immense energy, lying mostly dormant at the base of the spine. This energy is known as **Kundalini.** (Note: sex-energy is part of this power.) Full flowering of this energy is blocked by the **sex knot**. The **sex knot** is experienced at the level of the emotional heart due to feeling sexual impulses in the "heart" during an attractive response. The transcendence of this sex knot allows further progress and inward evolution. (Note: This transcendence of this sex knot does not mean denying sexual pleasure, as per the left-handed path.) The urge to procreate and other instinctual desires exist naturally. In Eastern spiritual traditions, this sex knot is considered to be at the level of the root center (**muladhara**) and the sex-center (**swadhistana**). Fear and potent pleasure concentrate sex energy and strengthen these psychological blocks/knots. In most people, sex energy is fragmented in many ways due to consciousness being held at this level. The holding of consciousness at this level occurs due to basic instincts of sexuality, sensuality, procreation, urge to survive, etc., given that survival of the human species depends upon it. The complete untying or dissolution of the sex knot is entrance into stage 7 where sexual pleasure is subjectively experienced and perceived only as a limited experience of unending ecstasy. There is a pronounced transition from erotic functioning of the human brain to ecstatic functioning of the entire neuropsychological system.

> ***Pleasure is like a drop of water and ecstatic love is like the ocean. – Sachin J. Karnik***

The Life Force (Prana) and the Little Death (In Men):

According to several Eastern spiritual traditions, sex energy is considered to be part of a greater energy known as **prana**. **Prana** is an abundant storehouse of energy that flows within each person. The term "**prana**" is a **Sanskrit** term that refers to one's life force or vital energy, which permeates the body and is especially concentrated along the midline in the **chakras**.

The **chakras** can be perceived in deep meditation as spinning vortices that link the mind with the spiritual dimension. There are 7 major chakras that have been described in yoga literature: 1) **Muladhara** (Root Chakra); 2) **Swadhistana** (Sex Energy Chakra); 3) **Manipura** (Navel Chakra); 4) **Anahata** (Heart Chakra); 5) **Vishuddhi** (Throat Chakra); 6) **Ajna** (A Two-Petal Lotus between the eyebrows); 7) **Sahasrara** (Crown Chakra); a 1000-petal lotus, that once opened, takes the spiritual aspirant into the spiritual dimension, beyond physical reality). These 7 chakras as well as various spiritual nerves (**nadis**) that flow through and around them can be perceived in deep meditation only. There is no physical way to prove these 7 chakras exist. Thousands of years ago in India, extensive spiritual research took place where mystics engaged in deep meditation to find out what exists within the "inner world." They perceived these non-physical vortices and found spiritual nerves called **nadi**(s) that connect the **chakras** together. It is estimated that around 72 thousand **nadis** exist within the human body connecting all 7 **chakras**. Additionally, the mystics are said to have discovered that chakras have abundant energy flowing in them and are lit by the light of the spiritual self (**atma**, or **soul**) within. All this is quite mystically wondrous and is a matter of personal spiritual exploration. In this meditative exploration, one can discovery for oneself what happens when energies are conserved and sublimated into refined mental/emotional/spiritual power. This refined power is known as **ojas**.

Prana is a great force that runs through these chakras where sex energy is *the* core energy that exists within **prana**. Hence, the energy used in formation of orgasmic experiences has much to do with usage and revitalization of **prana**. In fact, in an ancient naturalistic medicine system known as "*Ayurveda,*" the term **prana** refers to natural psychosexual energies that can be used to heal the body by its own energy. **Prana** also refers to energy in breathing because breath is integral within one's "life force" sustaining the whole body. **Prana** is considered to be the sun's energy that has been transferred into food and then into the form of one's body. While in the body, the sex energy is the creative force of **prana** and is at the core of **prana.** For the purposes of discussion in this book, all the following terms are used synonymously: **prana, sex energy, orgasmic energy, neuropsychic energy, neurophysiological energy, root energy, and psycho-emotive energy.** Although there are differences in the way each of these is conceptualized based on scientific terminology, spiritual practices, or cultural notions, the intention is to increase awareness of this great energy existing within oneself. **Energy is only ONE**. It takes various forms such as: sexual energy, emotional energy, cognitive energy, physiological energy, dream-state energy, etc. At the root of all these expressions of energy is undifferentiated energy experienced as "sex energy" fundamental to life.

With this brief background, we can consider **prana** to be one's stored reservoir of energy. It is believed in Eastern psycho-sexual traditions that men use a large portion of **prana** during ejaculatory orgasm. If this energy is conserved by using either tantric methods (i.e. combining meditation with sexual stimulation) or non-sexual meditation paths, then this energy remains stored within the mind/brain in the form of **ojas**. **Ojas** is sublimated sex energy that has remarkable potential in increasing mental vigor, physical stamina, and can possibly open the spiritual dimension of one's own being. As part of yoga practice (tantric sex practices or non-sexual practices), the goal of **yogis** (those individuals who are attempting to sublimate their sexual energies and connect with the spiritual dimension) is to prevent the loss of **prana** (via loss of sexual energies) and store as much **ojas** as possible. This storehouse of **ojas** can lead to a state of enlightenment that is described in stage 7 as a state of absolute and unending non-directional ecstasy, compassion, and undiluted love.

(Just to clarify further, the conservation of sexual energies in men occurs through the conservation of semen, and this conservation is part of the **urdhvareeta** (i.e. upward flow of semen) state of functioning. **Ojas**, for men, is the transmuted form of the "gross semen" where energies that are usually lost in ejaculatory orgasm are conserved and transformed into a highly refined form of potent spiritual energy. This term "**Ojas**" is a Sanskrit term that was developed by ancient Hindu sages thousands of years ago. They stated that sex energy is a significant part of Divine power or the power of God that runs throughout the universe in various forms. They also discovered that sublimation/conservation of this energy has incredible potential to open a gateway into the spiritual dimension of reality. Before this spiritual dimension opens up, there are intermediate stages where psychological blocks, emotional problems, and internal/external conflicts must fall away naturally due to the power of sex sublimation. This is not to say that men who are having the usual ejaculatory orgasm cannot remove these blocks by non-sexual means. There are many non-sexual meditation methods aimed at removing **psychological blocks**. Even in those methods, it is sex energy is the stabilized and harmonized within oneself. With regards to women, **ojas** is also sex energy that has been sublimated and transformed where multi-orgasmic experiences are an intermediate stage of development for greater mastery over the sex energy and its possible sublimation.)

It should be noted that many spiritual traditions in the West also place emphasis on conservation of sex energy. Irrespective of Western or Eastern traditions, conservation of sex energy has potential physical, mental, and emotional health benefits due to the storage of energy and the intelligent use of this energy. In the French language there is the expression, "**le petit mort**" meaning the "little death," which is considered to be male ejaculation. This is not, of course, actual death. It merely expresses the fact that a great amount of neurophysiological and psycho-emotive energy is used in the ejaculatory orgasm. This use of energy is considered depletion, to some extent, of male vitality and a temporary extinguishing of desire or pleasure. This neurophysiological and psycho-emotive energy is part of what the Eastern spiritualists call **prana**, as discussed earlier. The entire practice of tantric sex (for men) is based on the man holding the key to managing his ejaculatory orgasm, because it is the man who experiences the greatest loss of sex energy (**prana)**. For men, overall physical, mental, spiritual vibrancy and liveliness are linked to the conservation, transformation, and sublimation of sex energy. The "little death" can be considered as an induced state where pleasure is decreased along with depletion of male vitality. This significant reduction or "draining" of pleasure is natural, given the dynamics of the sexual response cycle. It should be reiterated that there is nothing wrong with the "usual ejaculatory orgasm." The intention of the writer is to point out that men generally want greater sexual pleasure and are frequently trying to find ways to increase it or sustain it. Hence, the methods of tantric (meditative) sexual practices can open the door to increased pleasure, repetitive orgasmic experiences, and conservation of energies, all at the same time.

Before the importance/significance of sex energy sublimation can be fully understood or accepted, consider the fact that ejaculatory orgasm has as its effect, a significant loss of pleasure after experiencing a powerful peak of pleasure. This can be considered as a depletion of male vitality. If one disagrees with this, then that is absolutely fine. The intention/purpose of the author is to encourage readers to directly see *if* this is true for oneself. Note that the amount of depletion of energy various considerable among men.

Having said that, let's continue the exploration of the "little death." Many **yogis** believe that the storehouse of **prana** (life force) is in the pelvis area and it is an enormous amount of life force energy. They also state that the amount of **prana** one can expel is limited, and it is very difficult to become spiritually vibrant by expelling large amounts of sex energy. For women, this is also true to some extent, but not to the same amount. In Eastern traditions, many spiritual masters were studying sexual processes as a means to understand the effects of these processes on physical health. These masters of sex energy believed that ejaculation caused significant reduction in a man's energy, increase in fatigue, increased desire for sleep, and possible weight gain. Many men, after ejaculating, find greater comfort with a blanket or pillows rather than with their partner due to desire being extinguished leading to loss of pleasure and reduction in overall energy level. (This experience is sometimes described in some spiritual texts as a "cool" state of mind that results from the drain of energy. The "hot" state of mind is considered to be the peak of ejaculatory orgasm.) From this perspective, ejaculatory orgasm can be conceptualized as a brief and potent state of pleasure (sensation) that brings with it a longing for sleep, weakness within the body, and overall tiredness. Even in the Western world, the importance of sex energy conservation can be seen by the following examples:

1) Many athletes will abstain from sexual activity for several days before playing a very important game or competing in an athletic event.
2) Many musicians will abstain from sexual activity for several days before a big concert.
3) Male astronauts will refrain from ejaculatory orgasms for a certain period before their missions.

Note that many young men may not notice a significant state of reduction of energy unless they are exerting themselves or are physically ill. This is due to hormonal levels as well as other physiological factors. Physical illness or some chronic health problems already cause a reduction in energy levels. When ejaculatory orgasms occur, there is possibly, further deterioration of overall health in individuals who already have an illness. Once again, this is a matter of personal experience and should not be considered as applicable to everyone. In general, we can conjecture that most men experience great difference in energy level reduction between: a) orgasms without ejaculation, and b) orgasms with ejaculation. In many cultures, it is assumed that the peak of male sexual arousal and the end of lovemaking is an ejaculatory orgasm in men. One of the major goals of the tantric (meditative) sexual practices is for the lovemaking to continue even after the lovemaking session has ended. This is possible if men are able to separate orgasmic pleasure from ejaculation and tap into the possibility of recirculating pleasure without losing the movement of pleasure as is usually the case when a man ejaculates.

In probing the nature of ejaculation, a bit further, please consider the following:

a) Ejaculation can be exhausting to one's body, to some extent or another in men.
b) An average ejaculation contains 50 to 250 million sperm cells.
c) Each sperm cell has the capacity to create ½ of a new human being.
d) If energies that are required to produce sperm cells (or the overall ejaculate) can be conserved, then this energy has the potential to improve one's physical and emotional health, stimulate and expand creative energies, and possibility open a gateway to the spiritual dimension.
e) It is possible to conceptualize that the male body is attempting to create a new life when ejaculation occurs. This could imply that various glands, organs, tissues, and cells in the body are releasing "high quality energy." This energy becomes concentrated and is experienced as **orgasmic energy**.

Orgasmic energy is a highly concentrated type of energy present in the experience of sexual pleasure. Sexual pleasure is sought after intensely and repeatedly due to the momentary non-dual experience of orgasm where polarity of male and female becomes ONE.

-- Sachin J. Karnik

For Women:

The "Sex-Orgasm-Celibacy Continuum" for women is depicted below:

FIGURE 6
SEX-ORGASM-CELIBACY (BRAHMACHARYA) CONTINUUM FOR WOMEN

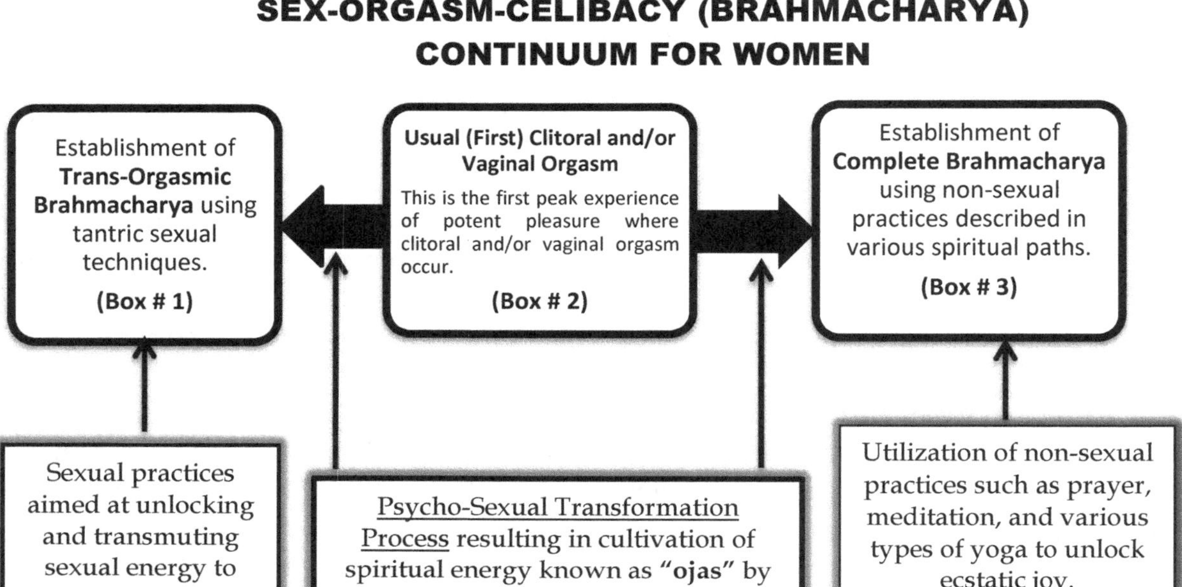

The "**Sex-Orgasm-Celibacy Continuum**" is, of course, as equally relevant for women as it is for men. In examining the continuum shown above (Figure 6), we can see that transformative processes occur by women experiencing multiple orgasms if using meditative sex practices. A major difference between men and women in box # 2 is that women generally do not have the same level of drain in sexual energy (**prana** = life force) and reduction in desire as experienced by men in the refractory period after having an ejaculatory orgasm. Thus, it is possible for women to have multiple clitoral and/or vaginal orgasms and whole-body orgasms without experiencing the type of refractory period men experience after ejaculation. Female ejaculation is also possible based on a variety of physical and psychological factors. Many women can have orgasms with minimal sexual fluid discharge.

There is, of course, a refractory period after any orgasm for women, yet there is not a significant dropping of desire and sexual energy as is in men. Once women experience multiple orgasms, they may come to the point of experiencing a "final orgasm" and enter into a refractory period that is similar to the refractory period in men, where there is absence of further desire for sexual stimulation and a sense of deep satisfaction. This is illustrated in figure 7 shown below.

FIGURE 7
(MEDITATIVE SEXUAL PRACTICES FOR WOMEN)

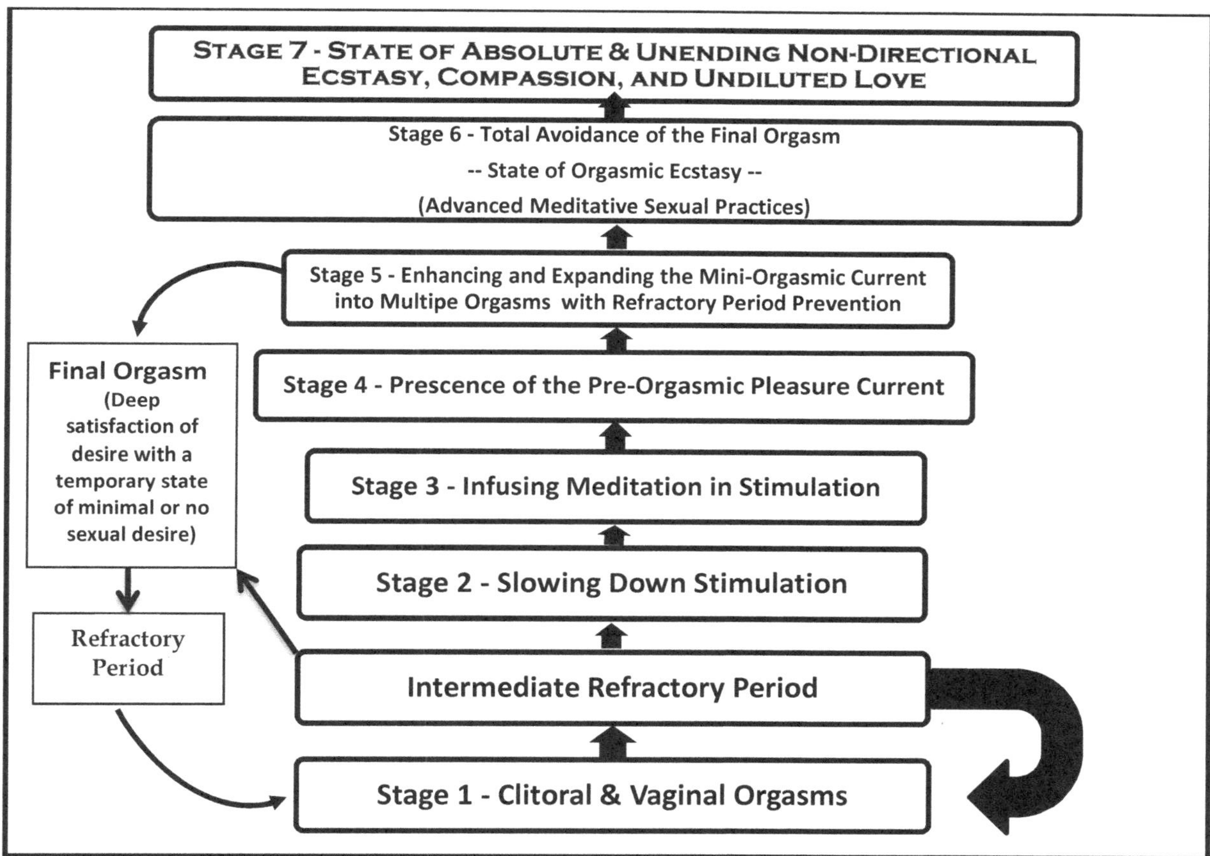

As it can be expected, there are some stark differences in the nature of sexual activity in stages 1-6 compared to male practices. The figure above gives an overview of 7 stages that describe the transformative processes that occur in the continuum for women. A brief examination of these stages is discussed below.

- **Stage 1**: During this stage, there is stimulation of female sexual organs leading to clitoral and/or vaginal orgasms. Also, the overall female body can be much more erotic than the male body. In the male body, there generally is not the same type of erotic experience by rubbing areas of the skin as there is in the female body.

Again, this is a matter of personal experience to determine the location of erogenous zones.

- **Intermediate Refractory Period**: Once the first clitoral and/or vaginal orgasm occurs, women do enter into a refractory period, yet, they are able to resume further stimulation and have another clitoral and/or vaginal orgasm. It is possible to have multiple orgasms this way, just moving from stage 1 to the intermediate refractory period, back to stage 1 where further stimulation leads to another orgasm. It should also be noted that the amount of **prana** lost during the intermediate refractory period is substantially less compared to men entering into the refractory period after an ejaculatory orgasm. This minimal loss of **prana** (life-force) allows women to have multiple orgasms.

- After experiencing multiple orgasms, many women may experience a "final orgasm" or what may be better called as a "**female peak orgasm**" with pronounced satisfaction of sexual desire and deep satiety (i.e. further stimulation is not desired) leading into a post-orgasmic refractory period. Deep gratification results with a temporary state of minimal or no desire for further sexual stimulation. In figure 7, the box entitled, "refractory period" refers to this state of minimal desire, a state of satisfaction of deep rooted sexual impulses, and an overall sense of great fulfillment. This is very natural; however, there are many women who do not experience this level of fulfillment with their male partners. Male partners may be satisfied sexually before the female partner experiences multiple orgasms. The final orgasm, as a climax point for women, may not occur at all due to male partner being satisfied via ejaculatory orgasm.

- **Stage 2:** If several orgasms have occurred, those women who are interested in using the sex energy for spiritual transformation can move into stage 2 where there is significant slowing down of stimulation. Slowing down is necessary in an attempt to become increasingly aware of the nature of orgasmic pleasure currents moving through the system. In this state, there can be greater emotional connection with one's partner, leading to greater mental openness that enhances intimacy.

- **Stage 3:** During this stage, infusion of meditation techniques brings greater stability to sex energy movement within the system. The crux of these techniques is to perform deep breathing to induce relaxation while orgasmic pleasure currents are moving through the system. (Again, this is covered in detail in Chapter 7.)

- **Stage 4:** If adequate slowing down and relaxation occur as stimulation is moving toward orgasm, a **mini-orgasmic pleasure current** will appear. This is also known as a **valley orgasm,** and it can also be present in women as in men. (See Chapter 7 for more details.)

- **Stage 5:** It is possible for women to enhance and expand **mini-orgasmic pleasure currents** where they can eventually have whole-body orgasms with minimal loss of **prana**. These orgasms are much more powerful than the usual clitoral or vaginal orgasms. These orgasms can potentially clear emotional blocks and have many other wonderful effects. The key in stage 5 is for women to prevent the "final orgasm" that generally has significant loss of energy (**prana**), loss of desire, and an experience of deep satisfaction. If one is aiming for this final orgasm and is not aiming to go further toward spiritual realization, that is a matter of personal choice. Of course, experiencing the final orgasm is not necessarily a hindrance to further sex energy cultivation. It can serve to bring balance in female sexual desire and women can reengage in the entire process after the refractory period ends.

If further stimulation is performed slowly, either with a partner who knows the location of various erogenous zones on the female body or in solo masturbation mode, then it is possible to enter into a meditative state with greater awareness of the presence of pre-orgasmic currents of pleasure.

SEXUAL DESIRE & CUPID'S FIVE ARROWS OF SEX

There is tremendous power in sex. In Eastern traditions, Cupid is known as "**Kaam Dev,** a demi-god responsible for **libido**." This concept of a demi-god for libido refers to sexual energy centers in the body that have neuropsychological connections. There is a description in the Hindu tradition of Cupid's five arrows that attract men to women and women to men as follows:

Mohana – This refers to fascination that occurs in the minds of men or women when a beautiful form of the opposite sex is seen. Finding the source of this fascination is a matter of deeper inner reflection and meditation. One may ask, why does this fascination occur at all and what is meant by a "beautiful form" that <u>causes</u> such fascination/attraction? This fascination (**mohana**) has the capacity to move sexual energy in the male body where physiological changes can be detected. The mental aspects of fascination are very subtle and have great speed compared to physiological aspects. Meditation is required to unravel, from within oneself, the psychological production of fascination. The experience of **mohana** (fascination/attraction) can be a wonderful opportunity to dive deeper into one's own attractive response.

Stambhana - This refers to stupefaction that arrests one's attention. This process of stupefaction is extremely powerful when a man is attracted to a woman that he considers beautiful. The word "stupefaction" refers to an emotional state of overwhelming amazement. A state of amazement occurs as desire awakens to connect with the other person whom one finds attractive.

Unmadana - This refers to intoxication in that a person is deeply absorbed in the form of the other person. The deep absorption occurs where there is increased desire for connection and stimulation.

Soshana - This is a state of intense attraction that causes the semen in the male body to start moving. It is a "churning" of subtle neuropsychological energy. Semen is created by this "churning" process. Semen exists in subtle form throughout the male body and the attractive response creates a state of psychological and physiological emaciation where energy is pulled from other areas of the physical body and the mind.

Tapana—This refers to burning and inflaming of the emotional heart. This state occurs if there is rejection.

These five arrows are thrown into the male mind when he perceives a woman as attractive. It is nature's way of moving sex energy in the male body for the purpose of reproduction and, of course, the experience of orgasmic pleasure. Similar "arrows of desire" can be thrown by men on women, with obvious physiological differences.

Given that the "five arrows of cupid" are part of sexual desire, the nature of sexual desire needs to be examined. There are many synonyms for the word "**desire**" as follows: covet, crave, long for, need, aspire, ache, yearn, wish, request, plea, etc. There are also noun synonyms such as **motivation**, **lust**, **libido**, interest, **horniness**, **drive**, etc.[1]

All these words convey various aspects of sexual desire based on one's personal experience. Sexual desire has energy, intensity, and force that vary considerably from aversion to intense passion. Motivation is a substantial part of sexual desire with regards to the level of interest in sexual activity and amount of effort placed in obtaining sexual stimulation. Here are significant aspects of sexual desire:

1) **Motivation** exists as part of desire in general and gets focused with regards to sexual desire.

2) **Sexual attraction**, **libido**, and **lust** are similar ideas; yet, there are differences in the use of these three terms based on context. This context can be biological,

psychological, and social.

3) Levels of sexual desire vary considerable from person to person based on **hormonal levels**, level of disturbances in one's mind, contextual circumstances, and many other factors such as cultural norms, religious beliefs, etc.

4) One of the greatest commonalities in human life is sexual desire. It has a "language" of its own that transcends all human languages. Human languages attempt to describe this deeper "instinctual" force of sex that exists beyond language.

5) There are many inner and outer signals that can trigger sexual desire. Sexual desire along with the experience of pleasure is one of the most wonderful examples of **qualia**. **Qualia** is one's direct experience and is conceptualized as the "internal and subjective component of sense perceptions, arising from stimulation of the senses by phenomena." In the area of "**philosophy of mind,**" many philosophers describe **qualia** as ineffable, intrinsic, and private where experience occurs only directly. Consider the following: Is the sweetness of sugar within the sugar or does sugar trigger dormant sweetness that is already within oneself (i.e. the brain/mind)? Is the experience of sweetness merely a chemical reaction that is triggered by sugar in the mouth, and then subsequent reactions occur in other nerves in the brain where the brain generates the experience of sweetness? Is the experience of sweetness possible without consciousness (i.e. soul, **atma**, spirit) that is the **experiencer**? Without an **experiencer**, how can there be any experience at all? Or, is subjective experience merely an illusion as argued by some philosophers? These are deep questions indeed and worthy of much consideration given that sexual stimulation is a matter of direct and personal experience. Cupid's five arrows, as already discussed, are a matter of direct experience. **Qualia**, with regard to sexual stimulation, is the direct experience of sexual energy moving within oneself due to forces of desire seeking pleasure and gratification. Any attempt to communicate about one's own experience of sexual stimulation is utterly pale compared to the *actuality* of the experience. Hence, there is an ineffable quality to sexual experience where linguistic expressions and descriptions are inadequate. Any description of sexual stimulation is NOT the direct and non-verbal state of being in a state of stimulation. To move out of limited linguistic descriptions and increase awareness of the nature of one's own sexual energy and how the mind creates orgasmic experiences, *is* **qualia** with regard to one's sexuality. The ineffable nature of sexual stimulation refers to the fact that it is a matter of one's direct experience. There are deeply intrinsic aspects of the movement of sexual energy where this movement is extremely personal and can

be felt directly. Although the stimulation of sexual energy is dependent upon various stimuli, the flow of sexual energy and experience of sexual pleasure is intrinsic within oneself. These experiences are also intrinsically private due to being instantaneously comprehensible within one's consciousness.[2]

6) Sexual desire is a subjective and direct state of "wanting" experience that is triggered by internal and external cues. Awareness of the *nature of desire* is possible when direct inner perception of cues occurs. Cues are signals and indicators of the entire triggering process that are occurring neuropsychologically.

7) Imagination and fantasy are involved in activation of sexual desire. This occurs when perceiving an individual whom one finds attractive. An attractive response occurs subjectively, triggering neurophysiological changes. Imagination and fantasy are mentally generated and change the functioning of the brain. It could also be said that imagination and fantasy are emergent properties of the brain. Emergent entities or properties "arise" out of more fundamental entities, yet, are "novel" or "irreducible" with respect to them. Hence, imagination and fantasy with regards to sexual stimulation can be considered as emerging from the brain, which is a physical (material) entity.

8) Sexual desire and sexual tension are interrelated. Sexual tension develops when one has not had sexual stimulation for a certain period. When two individuals interact, there can be sexual tension although consummation may be postponed or may never occur. There can be physical attraction without any emotional attraction where sexual desire functions within that range only.

9) There is a dynamic nature to sexual desire and the intensity of desire varies based on the level of attractive response one has for any individual. Sexual desire exists in diverse ways and the type of response also exists in multiple ways as follows[3]:

   a) *Passion* — a deep attractive response that has increased sexual appetite.
   b) *Need* — a type of sexual release that is biological driven. This is at a lower level than passion.
   c) *Interest* — a level of possible attraction based on limited characteristics of another person.
   d) *Indifference* — a sexual response that is neutral without attraction or any aversion.
   e) *Disinclination* — a response that is lower than "indifference" where there is a non-attractive response.

f) *Aversion* – sexual dislike toward another person due to the person lacking desired characteristics.

10) Sexual desire can manifest itself with certain physical actions such as licking, sucking, puckering, touching the lips, and tongue protrusion.[4]

Please reflectively consider the following statements about the nature of desire:

- Desire is the lack of satisfaction. When desire is satisfied, desire *temporarily* does not exist. Sexual desire has a transient nature that produces transient fulfillment.
- Without desire, there cannot be any activity in life.
- The energy *within* desire can be used intelligently.
- Observation of desire leads to natural revitalization of the energy within desire.
- The wanting of sexual pleasure is a deep-seated desire within the human mind that has great energy. Realization of the relationship among desire, energy, emotions, thoughts, and actions leads to freedom.
- Desire creates friction and excitement. Energy is used in frictional excitement.
- Dropping the problems of the past, psychologically, is revitalization of positive desires in the present.
- Worry about the future is focused desire that destroys potency in the present.
- Once desires are non-contradictory within oneself, energy becomes harmonious.
- Clarity about what one wants in life is rare in most people. Energy revitalization can set the foundation for this clarity.
- Desire and thought are related. The existence of thought depends on desire.
- Freedom "from" desire and freedom "in" desire is quite different. To be completely free in the exploration of sexuality requires one to be psychologically free to explore the nature of one's own sexual desires. This freedom comes from observing and exploring without bias. Internal sexual conflicts can occur due to emotional blocks that are preventing freedom from flowering within oneself. What is the difference between "freedom from sexual desire" versus "freedom in sexual desire?"
- Pleasure and fear are deeply rooted within the psyche of each person. Desire is at the root of pleasure and fear. Energy is used in pleasure and fear due to desire moving in a direction. Sexual desire moves in a direction toward gratification.
- To fight with sexual pleasure is to strengthen it. To run after sexual pleasure excessively is to destroy creative energy.
- Inward meditation opens awareness of the "structure of desire." This structure is extremely subtle and exists within one's personality framework. Freedom from one's own limited view of sexual desire sets the foundation for inward exploration of the nature of sexual desire.

- Pleasure is based on memory of past enjoyments. Desire and pleasure are interdependent and cyclical.

  Please see the diagram below that shows how core energy exists within desire. This energy is the sex energy that works in diverse ways to activate thoughts and gives power to emotions. This same core energy is used to access memories. The diagram below shows that it is this core energy that functions *through* desire and interacts with actions, thoughts, emotions, and memories.

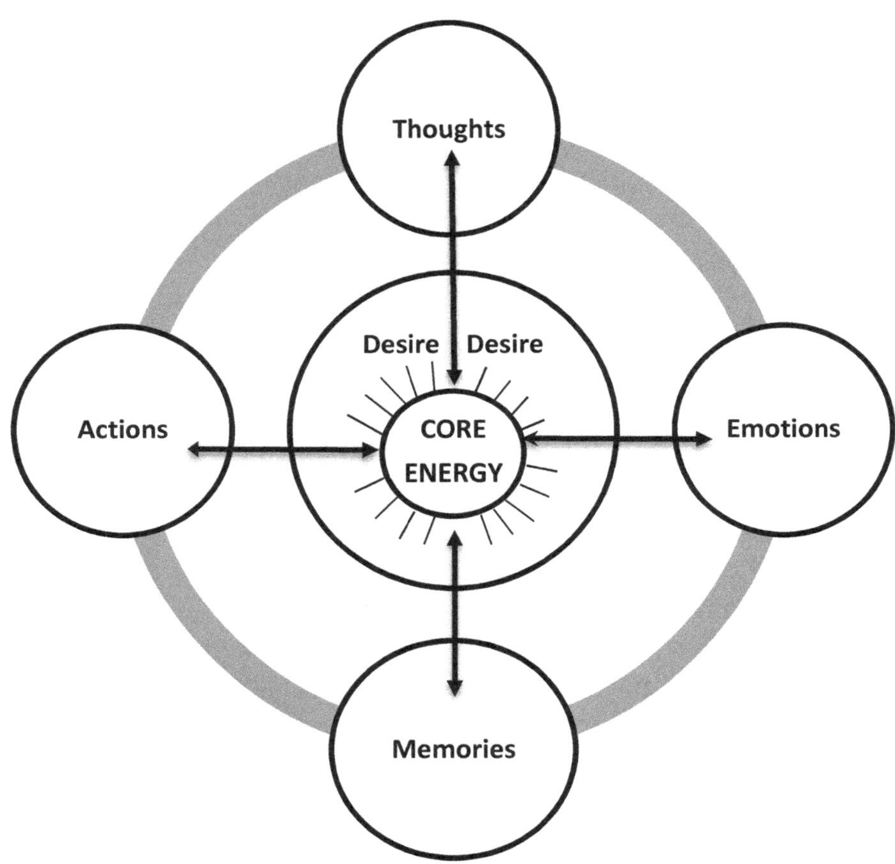

CHAPTER 4

CONTROL OF SEXUAL ENERGY

Controlling sex energy is the most perplexing task for the mind. Swinging of the mind between two poles of control vs. indulgence creates a tremendous inner war. Most of humanity is psychologically stuck in this inner war. Who is the winner and the loser of this war?
-- Dr. Sachin Karnik

SEX ENERGY TRANSFORMATION
(The Path of Control — A Warrior's Path)

Throughout the history of the world, various religious and spiritual paths have advocated for the ideal of transforming sexual energy for the purpose of **enlightenment**. In each of the major religions of the world (Judaism, Christianity, Islam, Buddhism, Hinduism, etc.) there is considerable emphasis placed on the observance of at least *some form* of **sexual continence** or restricted sex for the purpose of enlightenment. Before we get into a detailed discussion of sexual continence, it is necessary to examine briefly what is meant by the term "enlightenment." Enlightenment, in most spiritual traditions, refers to a state of profound clarity, total bliss, complete freedom from ignorance, etc. Fundamentally, it refers to a state of inner unfolding where **God** (or the **Ultimate Reality**) is directly perceived and experienced. In pursuing a state of enlightenment, most spiritual traditions have historically placed considerable emphasis on conserving sexual energies for the purpose of performing spiritual practices aimed at Self or God Realization. In the beginning of this book, we examined the nature of sex and normal functions of sex. Well, one may ask, why have so many spiritual paths from religions throughout the world placed emphasis on conservation of sexual energy (i.e. sexual continence, celibacy, or some level of restricted sexual function)? In the opinion of the author, the major reason is the recognition of the importance of sexual energy and its role in trying to connect with the Divine. *(Just as a reminder, please note that in this book, the word "divine" is used to mean: God, the soul, the spiritual dimension of one's being, super conscious state, the transcendental state of realization, and/or the solidification of truth-bliss-consciousness.)*

The next section, "why conserve sex energy" will be useful for the following readers:

a) Readers who are interested in using non-sexual approaches to achieve a state of complete sex energy transformation.
b) Readers who are curious about what is involved in non-sexual practices yet are more interested in sexual techniques for sex energy sublimation.

WHY CONSERVE SEX ENERGY?

When we examine many spiritual traditions, we find that in some form or another, there is emphasis placed on restricting sexual activity. The following questions easily come to mind regarding sexual restrictions:

1) **Why should sexual activity be restricted at all?**
2) **What is wrong with just engaging in and enjoying "normal sexual activities" that are naturally occurring in each human being?**
3) **Why is sexual pleasure considered to be an obstacle to enlightenment (God Realization, etc.)?**
4) **What's wrong with having as many ejaculations and orgasms as possible in life? Given that life is short, why not enjoy sexual pleasures to the highest extent?**
5) **Why is it necessary to become established in Brahmacharya, (i.e. conservation of sexual energies) and what is the significance of semen conservation in men and orgasmic transformation in women?**

These are extremely important questions and examining possible answers to these questions is critical before progress can be made in understanding the "**warrior's path**" aimed at sex sublimation. Let's examine each question, one at a time.

Question # 1: Why should sexual activity be restricted at all? This question is nearly universal in that most people have asked it, and there is usually some degree of frustration at the notion of the restriction of sex, since sex gives so much pleasure. As we stated before, each human being is in search of endless bliss, and sexual processes within a person provide an experience of concentrated pleasure that temporarily pulls one out of the mundaneness of day-to-day life. So, why have cultures, societies, religions, etc. placed restrictions on sex? There are many possible answers to this question, such as:

a) Creation and preservation of a family structure.
b) Development of greater emotional bond between man and woman.
c) Creation of the marriage system to provide:
    a. mutual security
    b. deeper emotional bonding
    c. care and safety of children
    d. providing support to members of the extended family
d) Prevention of teenage pregnancy.
e) Prevention of sexually transmitted diseases.
f) REcognition of the importance of conservation of sexual energies.
g) Recognition that heavy losses of semen (in men) can be a cause of:
    a. health problems
    b. reduction in thinking power

c. reduction in emotional sensitivity
d. increased desire for extra-marital affairs
e. increased need for additional sexual stimulation to achieve an ejaculatory orgasm
f. increased viewing of pornographic materials that takes one away from actual sexual relationship with a partner, where fantasy becomes psychologically more important in achieving sexual excitation and arousal, then sex without pornography.

Given these reasons for restricting sexual activity, cultures and religions over thousands of years have placed, to varying degrees, certain restrictions. These restrictions vary considerably and have a broad range.

Question # 2: What is wrong with just engaging in and enjoying the "normal sexual activities" that are naturally occurring in each human being?

There is absolutely nothing wrong with "normal sexual activity" and going through the sexual response cycle on a regular basis. Nonetheless, some adherents of various spiritual traditions are intent upon controlling sexual impulses and redirecting them toward the Divine (i.e. God, Higher Reality, etc.) for the purpose of enlightenment. There have been many aspirants on spiritual paths who believe that loss of sexual energy, via orgasm and ejaculations (in men), is a major setback on the spiritual path.

Question # 3: Why is sexual pleasure considered to be an obstacle to enlightenment (God Realization, etc.)?

Sexual pleasures are considered by certain spiritual paths to be obstacles to enlightenment because sexual pleasure is considered, in such paths, as a frictional process that uses energy needed for spiritual practices. It is the contention of these spiritual paths that a great deal of energy is required to establish a connection with the transcendental reality (i.e. God, the Divine, the Infinite, etc.), and this energy is expended by the activation, pursuit, and fulfillment of sexual desires.

Question # 4: What's wrong with having as many ejaculations and orgasms as possible in life? Given that life is short, why not enjoy sexual pleasures to the highest extent?

In any spiritual tradition that emphasizes the need to control sexual desire, prominence is placed on the need to prevent sexual arousal so that orgasms do not occur. This has been emphasized due to the belief that in ejaculatory orgasm (men), there is much loss of psychological energy that needs to be used for deeper contemplation, concentration, and focus on a specific spiritual path. Sexual arousal has been considered by many spiritual paths to be a hindrance in realizing God. Hence, the following restrictions in many traditions have been placed on sexual activity:

1) No sex before marriage
2) No masturbation
3) No extra-marital affairs
4) No viewing of pornographic materials
5) Have sexual contact only for the purpose of having children

Question # 5: Why is it necessary to become established in Brahmacharya (i.e. conservation of sexual energies) and what is the significance of semen conservation in men and orgasmic transformation in women?

The significance of the conservation of sex energy, via semen conservation in men and sexual essences sublimation in women, is emphasized in many spiritual paths. Eleven major reasons for the conservation of sex energy, *according to many spiritual paths that advocate non-sexual sex-sublimation techniques*, are shown below:

1) In some theories about sex energy, heavy losses of semen cause a reduction in the average life of men. According to various yoga traditions, it is believed that men can live 100 years if there is adequate conservation of semen. It can be hypothesized that conservation has great health benefits due to energy being harnessed for the purpose of meditation and serving society.

2) Complete eradication of lust and becoming established in mental **Brahmacharya** (i.e. sex energy conservation) lead to direct realization of one's own spiritual self (i.e. the holy spirit, **atma, Akshara, Parabrahma**, etc.) Great forces of sexual desire are located in the minds of human beings for the purpose of propagation of the species and for redirection of this force back to its origin, where this redirection results in opening a doorway into the kingdom of God (i.e. **moksha**, etc.).

3) Enduring the force of sexual desire and potent passion can lead to great harmony and happiness in one's life.

4) Engaging in sexual acts in any form and via any means creates what is known as a "**Samskara**" or impressions in the subconscious mind (i.e. **chitta**). These impressions are neurological processes where "neurons that fire together, wire together." These psychological impressions raise what is known as a "thought wave" (**vrutti**) and this "thought wave" again creates additional impressions. The physical semen (**veerya**) is the essence of a complex psycho-physical process that is the quintessential essence of blood. In an ancient medical tradition known as "*Ayurveda*" it is contended that it takes 40 drops of blood to create 1 drop of semen.

5) The physical body is considered to have **7 essences** (**dhatus**) where semen is considered to be the last essence formed out of food. The seven essences are listed below:

    - From food, chyle is manufactured. "**Chyle** is a milky bodily fluid consisting of lymph and emulsified fats or free fatty acids (FFAs). It is formed in the small intestine during digestion of fatty foods, and taken up by lymph vessels specifically known as lacteals. The relative low pressure of the lacteals allows large fatty acid molecules to diffuse into them, whereas the higher pressure in veins allows only smaller products of digestion, like amino acids and sugars, to diffuse into the blood directly."[1]

- From chyle, **blood** is formed. "Blood is a bodily fluid in animals that delivers necessary substances such as nutrients and oxygen to cells and transports metabolic waste products away from those same cells. In vertebrates, it is composed of blood cells suspended in blood plasma. Plasma, which constitutes 55% of blood fluid, is mostly water (92% by volume), and contains dissipated proteins, glucose, mineral ions, hormones, carbon dioxide (plasma being the main medium for excretory product transportation), and blood cells themselves. Albumin is the main protein in plasma, and it functions to regulate the colloidal osmotic pressure of blood. Blood cells are mainly red blood cells (also called RBCs or erythrocytes) and white blood cells, including leukocytes and platelets. The most abundant cells in vertebrate blood are red blood cells. These contain hemoglobin, an iron-containing protein, which facilitates transportation of oxygen by reversibly binding to this respiratory gas and greatly increasing its solubility in blood. In contrast, carbon dioxide is almost entirely transported extracellularly dissolved in plasma as bicarbonate ion."[2]

- **Blood** contains the basic nutrients to create muscle tissue. From blood and muscle tissue, bones are created. "Bones are rigid organs that constitute part of the endoskeleton of vertebrates. They support and protect the various organs of the body, produce red and white blood cells and store minerals. Bone tissue is a type of dense connective tissue. Bones come in a variety of shapes and have a complex internal and external structure, are lightweight, yet strong and hard, and serve multiple functions. One of the types of tissue that makes up bone is the mineralized osseous tissue, also called bone tissue, that gives it rigidity and a coral-like three-dimensional internal structure. Other types of tissue found in bones include marrow, endosteum, periosteum, nerves, blood vessels and cartilage. At birth, there are over 270 bones in an infant human's body, but many of these fuse together as the child grows, leaving a total of 206 separate bones in a typical adult, not counting numerous small sesamoid bones and ossicles. The largest bone in the human body is the femur and the smallest bone of the 206 is the stapes."[3]

- "**Bone marrow** is the flexible tissue in the interior of bones. In humans, red blood cells are produced by cores of bone marrow in the heads of long bones in a process known as hematopoiesis. On average, bone marrow constitutes 4% of the total body mass of humans; in an adult weighing 65 kilograms (143 lb), bone marrow typically accounts for approximately 2.6 kilograms (5.7 lb). The hematopoietic component of bone marrow produces approximately 500 billion blood cells per day, which use the bone marrow vasculature as a conduit to the body's systemic circulation. Bone marrow is also a key component of the lymphatic system, producing the lymphocytes that support the body's immune system."[4]

- **Semen** is created out of bone marrow.

6) **Semen** is considered the last **dhatu** as we have seen above. From food to **chyle**, from **chyle** to blood, from blood to flesh, from flesh to fat, from fat to bone, from bone to bone marrow, and finally, from bone marrow to semen. Please mark the *preciousness* of semen. The term "**dhatu**" refers to essence or precious substance. It is imperative to recognize that our entire body is created from food, and within the body these 7 **dhatus** are transformations of food based on one's genetic code. These seven **dahtus** are the support of one's physical body. Semen is the final essence and is the essence of essences. Semen is manufactured out of a complex series of biochemical processes and neuropsychological processes. The "falling of semen" is considered to be a "little death" (i.e. **la petite mort** in the French language) that is aimed at creating life. The preservation of semen brings tremendous vitality as it is *the* hidden treasure in the male body. The preservation and subsequent transformation has the capacity to impart what is known as "**brahma-Tejas**" (i.e. divine light) on the face of a man and can also bring great strength to one's intellect.

7) **Yogic masters**, who are considered to be proficient in the sublimation of semen, state that this vital fluid (i.e. semen) is reabsorbed in the body and transformed into divine energy known as "**ojas**." This is possible for those whose life is filled with purity and mental/physical discipline. This reabsorption gives tremendous strength to a man's body and mind while endowing him with purified emotion and thought. The excessive wastage of this fluid can leave a man feeling drained of energy, physically weak, prone to being increasingly irritated in many aspects of life, and causing difficulties in maintaining a sustained relationship with a significant other. Some spiritual masters even state that excessive loss of semen can lead to sexual disorders, a weak nervous system, diseases such as epilepsy, and many other physical/mental health problems.

8) There is a well-known statement about the conservation of sexual energies that states, *"If one practices celibacy for a period of twelve years by his thought, word and deed, then he is bestowed with the vision of God."* This vision of God is possible due to the full sublimation of sexual energy where it reaches its origin point. This origin point is God (i.e. Ultimate Reality, Universal Energy, etc.)

9) "Scientists have analyzed semen and found it to be amazingly rich in hormones, proteins, vitamins, minerals, ions, enzymes, trace elements, and other vital substances. By nature's arrangement, this substance, when mixed with the ovum, is sufficient for the procreation of a new body. By nature's arrangement also, if it is not used for procreation but is kept within, it nourishes the body and the brain in a way impossible for any tonic or dietary aid to emulate. The current craze for vitamin and mineral supplements is an attempt to make up for self-imposed deficiencies. Most people do not know that they are reducing their very life energy with that essential bodily fluid. If semen is lost, all bodily and sensory functions are weakened. Repeated loss of semen reduces storage of pure (**sattvika**) energy and utilization of pure intelligence that is vital for spiritual growth and evolution. However, if semen is retained in the body, there is the possibility of developing what *Ayurveda* refers to as **ojas** (i.e. vital spiritually transformed energy) that gives strength, luster, enhanced mental abilities, immunity to diseases, and slows the aging process."[5]

10) Conservation of sex energies involves redirecting these energies for purposes other than orgasmic experiences. This change in direction of sex energy away from orgasms can lead to a state of mind where the **brahmachari** (i.e. one who conserves sex energy) strives for excellence in multiple domains in life, filled with activity and meaningful relationships (non-sexual of course) while pursuing a virtuous life. This has a similar meaning to the Greek concept of arête (excellence).

11) **Brahmacharya** (i.e. sex energy conservation) has the power to clear underlying personality conflicts and bring about meaningful centering within oneself. The practice of **brahmacharya** has considerable similarity to the aims of psychotherapy with goals of "clearing conflicts" and resolving "personality complexes." Conservation of sex energies has the power to remove psychological/emotional conflicts and bring tremendous clarity within oneself. This is due to the wonderful possibility that sexual energies can culminate into a state of wholeness where contradictory mental and emotional activity ceases. This cessation of contradictory activity occurs due to the sublimation of sexual impulses. Hence, **brahmacharya** is a type of natural psychotherapy that an individual may give to oneself due to personal recognition, via exploration, that sex energy conservation has great physical and mental health benefits.

As a response to the importance of conservation of sex energy, many spiritual paths have emphasized the need to "control" sexual desire and sexual activity and thus, have devised diverse practices (**sadhana**) to either partially restrict sexual activity or completely restrict it in an attempt to fully sublimate sex energy.

AROUSAL & RESTRICTIONS

In any spiritual tradition that emphasizes the need to control sexual desire, most such traditions emphasize the need to prevent sexual arousal so that orgasm does not occur. This has been emphasized due to the strong possibility that in ejaculatory orgasm (men), there is much loss of psychological energy that is needed as "fuel" to be used for deeper contemplation, concentration, and focus on a specific spiritual path. Sexual arousal has been considered by many spiritual paths to be a hindrance in realizing God. Hence, many traditions have placed the following restrictions on sexual activity:

1) No sex before marriage
2) No masturbation
3) No extramarital affairs
4) No viewing of pornographic materials
5) Have sexual contact only for conception of children

> ***Restrictions on sexual activity and sexual stimulation can have the purpose of harnessing sex energy through control. Desire can either strengthen or weaken when it is controlled based on level of inner realization of the nature of desire.***
>
> ***-- Sachin J. Karnik***

THE CONTROLLER & THE CONTROLLED

Irrespective of specific religious traditions or spiritual paths, the fact is that *any type of sexual control* leads to a division between the "**controller**" and the "**controlled**." This means that one thought (the controller) is trying to gain control over other thoughts. The **controller** can be understood to include:

a) The deciding factor within the field of thoughts that decides to restrain sexual desire.
b) The culturally or religiously conditioned aspect of one's personality that considers loss of sexual energy to be an obstacle toward enlightenment.
c) Internally generated desire to gain control over sexual desire. This internally generated desire could be the result of conditioning of one's own inner force to consider loss of sexual energy as a serious obstacle toward enlightenment.

The "**controlled**" can be understood to include:

a) The vast force of deep-seated and potent sexual desire.
b) Desires and forces that are considered "**inner enemies**" (particularly, sex desire is considered in some spiritual traditions as an "inner enemy.")
c) The multitude of other thoughts and emotions that want to fulfill deep-seated desires.

Control of sexual energy is emphasized in many spiritual/religious traditions and paths with a goal of conserving sex energy and using it for spiritual practices (**sadhana**). Most individuals attempting to control sexual desire are also intent upon preventing the experience of orgasmic pleasures, and invariably find themselves in a battle with sexual desire. This inner battle is a natural consequence of the psychological division between the **controller** and the **controlled**. Nonetheless, this battle has immense value for anyone who is trying to conserve sex energies on this path. An individual going through such a battle gains deeper understanding and awareness about the *nature* of sexual desire itself. This can provide greater awareness about one's inner process of sexual desire formation. Hence, going through such a battle also has benefits to some extent.

A battle between the controller and the controlled can turn into a terrible inner war. The path of sublimating sex energy via control can bring awareness to the mind about the mind. It is a path filled with many pitfalls and inner struggles. Courage and patience are absolutely necessary to make progress on the path of control.

-- Sachin J. Karnik

FIGURE 8
THE CONTROLLER & THE CONTROLLED

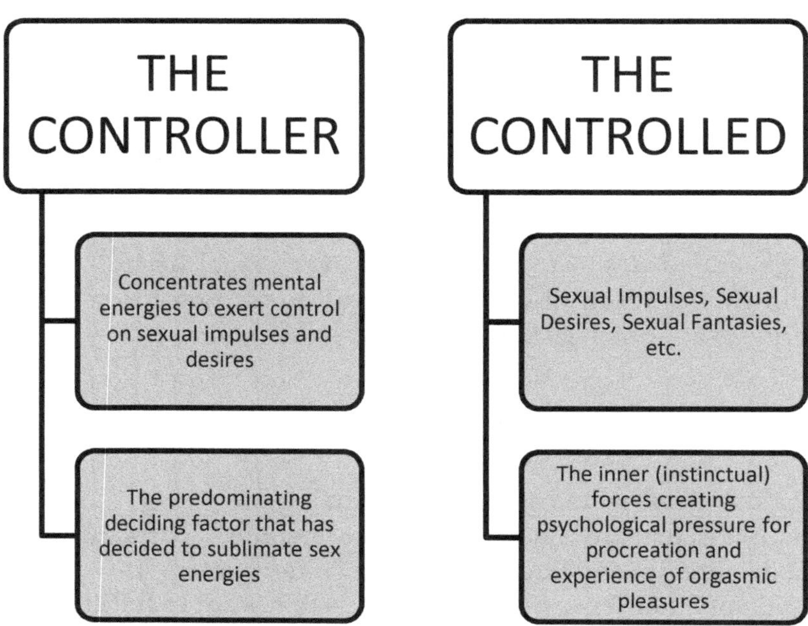

There is little doubt that profound psychological wars exist within most individuals who are trying to control their sexual desires. Control *implies* both a controller and the controlled. If this is clear, then let us consider what exactly is necessary to be successful in this "warrior's path of control." The author wants to make it *absolutely clear* that he is not against the path of control. In fact, it is a path that has been advocated by great spiritual teachers all over the world, and it is possible for spiritual aspirants **(sadhakas)** to progress well on this path. There are, of course, many unfortunate consequences if sufficient progress is not made on this path. Chapter 5 deals with these problems and how to resolve these difficulties. (Please note that the philosopher, **J. Krishnamurti,** has expounded upon the problem of "the controller" vs. "the controlled.")

The purpose of the "fight or internal war" is create a mental state where the fight ends completely. This can result in a full-blown flowering of spiritual unfoldment. In such a state, all psychological fragments combine in the wholeness of one's own being.

> ***When love flowers in its real sense, all battles end. Energy becomes whole.***
>
> ***-- Sachin J. Karnik***

BOUNDARIES PLACED ON SEXUAL ACTIVITY & EROTIC PLEASURE

There is quite a bit of emphasis placed on complete transcendence of sexual desires (i.e. sexual energy) in some religious/spiritual traditions. This may have to do with the level of experimentation performed with sexuality in these traditions. Interestingly, inner research of this type aims to introspectively and experientially unravel the origin of sexual processes with the aim of sex energy sublimation.

Various religious/spiritual teachers in the East and West have emphasized placing boundaries on sexual activity. Some of them have placed emphasis on sublimating sex energies. Various denominations, sects, and offshoots of various traditions advocate strict celibacy to severely limit sexual contact outside a pre-determined boundary of interaction. In Eastern and western spiritual traditions, teachers/masters/gurus placed varying degrees of emphasis on the conservation and sublimation of sexual desires, sexual impulses, and **sexual essences**. In examining this further, it can be seen (historically and at present) that boundaries have been placed on the act of sex in one or more of the following ways all over the world:

1) Sexual activity is controlled via the bonds of marriage or similar commitment to only one partner. (There are some exceptions to this in some traditions.)

2) **Adultery** is forbidden in many traditions. (It is considered either as sinful or as an act that creates great negative **karmic effects** and prevents an individual from connecting with the Divine.)

3) **Fornication** is also forbidden in many spiritual traditions. Fornication is premarital sexual intercourse, and this is considered to create an increase in sexual desires and a cause of marital instability and conflict. (Although most western cultures and many areas in the Eastern culture now accept fornication as irresistible, some spiritual leaders today still preach abstinence as the ideal state.)

4) In some orthodox and ultraconservative Eastern spiritual paths, male monks are to follow what is known as "**eightfold celibacy**" (***ashtanga-brahmacharya***), in an attempt to completely sublimate, transform, and redirect all sexual energy. This eight-fold path entails a monk to take the following vows as part of his vow of celibacy:
    a. not to deliberately look at a woman (control of eyes)
    b. not to deliberately hear the voice of a woman (control of ears)
    c. not to touch a woman of any age (control of sense of touch)
        i. If a deliberate touch occurs, then the monk is to fast without taking food or water the next day.

    ii. The monk must perform other deeper meditation practices to completely remove the possibility of orgasmic currents flowing through his system. This is done to prevent loss of sexual fluids via ejaculation, even in the dream state.

d. not to talk to a woman personally or by any other form of communication.
e. not to engage in conversations about women with others.
f. not to think about the form of a woman.
g. not to contemplate about the form of a woman and not to remember past sexual enjoyments.
h. Not to deliberately discharge one's semen by masturbation.

NON-SEXUAL SEX ENERGY SUBLIMATION TECHNIQUES

Some readers may be interested in sex energy sublimation techniques via non-sexual methods. The upcoming 27 dimensions of clear understanding are especially written for these readers. Nonetheless, it is beneficial for all readers to know what is involved in sex energy sublimation without utilizing the pre-orgasmic stimulation techniques shown later in this book. These non-sexual techniques are used by some spiritual practitioners to enter a state of total sex energy sublimation **(Brahmacharya)**. This is certainly no easy task and generally involves controlling desires, avoiding close contact with the opposite sex, and many other practices such as intense prayers, fasting, meditation, and inner contemplation.

The path of achieving a total transformation of one's sexual desires and sex energies by controlling them is a type of "**warrior's path**." This path has been attempted by many spiritual aspirants all over the world and many have tragically failed to *properly* sublimate their sexual energies, in the opinion of the author. Success in this "**warrior's path** — the path of control" is extremely rare. The path of control, which entails moving completely out of sexual pleasure, requires strict denial of sexual pleasure. Such denial is extremely difficult to practice, and is usually filled with strong negative side effects of long-term **suppression**. Suppression is a state of control of desire with the aim of preventing the experience of orgasmic pleasure. Control inherently implies a division between the **controller** and the **controlled**. This division creates **intrapsychic conflicts** and leads to much confusion, self-blame, and a deep sense of failure. Nonetheless, sublimation of sexual energies by suppressing them has been advocated by various spiritual/religious traditions and by many spiritual/religious teachers. If one is interested in following this path, the author discusses it starting on page 81. It is called the "**warrior's path**," because it is a path of control where one is fundamentally "at war" with one's natural instinctual drives. This war is played out in the mind of the "warrior" who is trying to prevent the triggering of orgasmic pleasure. The goal of sublimating sexual essences, via strict control, is an attempt to fully conserve energies that are normally lost during ejaculatory orgasm in men and the final orgasm in women. This "final orgasm" in women is when there is loss of desire for further orgasm.

Based on the author's extensive study of many spiritual traditions and paths, the following 27 dimensions[6] of clear understanding, clear vision, and sustained spiritual practices are required for any aspirant (**sadhaka**) interested in completely sublimating sexual energies and transforming them into refined forms (**ojas**):

1) He who has eradicated lust completely is constantly connected with the Divine. This requires developing and maintaining a lucid understanding of the importance of semen conservation. Three major practices are advocated to achieve semen conservation: a) keeping the mind engaged in activity related toward God, b) following strict rules about food intake, sleep, meditation, religious service, and other such practices, and c) balancing breathing via yogic breathing practices.

2) A sexual act produces an impression (i.e. a **samskara**) in the subconscious mind (**chitta**). This impression (**samskara**) raises a thought wave (**vritti**) in the mind and that thought wave again causes further impressions in the subconscious mind. This becomes a deepening cycle that strengthens desires.

3) **Semen** is considered the quintessence of blood. It is the final product of nutrients being processed in blood.

4) According to the yoga tradition, semen is the last essential substance (**dhatu**) that is formed out of food. **Chyle** is manufactured out of food and from **chyle** comes blood. Out of blood, flesh and fat are formed. Bones are also formed within which bone marrow is formed that ultimately creates semen. The semen is extremely precious.

5) Loss of semen reduces mental strength. Real vitality in men comes from semen conservation as it is the hidden treasure within each man. Conserved semen imparts what is known as "**Brahma-Tej**" (divine light) to the face and tremendous mental clarity and strength to the intellect.

6) The best blood in the body goes to form the elements of reproduction. Semen conservation leads to natural reabsorption of this vital fluid and is carried back into the neurophysiological system.

7) If semen is excessively wasted, it can leave a man effeminate, weak, physically debilitated, and increasingly prone to sexual irritation and possibly other health problems. If semen is conserved (without psychological suppression), it can provide notable increases in physical, mental, and spiritual vigor.

8) The mind, **prana** (breathing force), and semen (**veerya**) are three links of one chain. They are three pillars of the soul. If one destroys one pillar (i.e. mind, prana, or semen), then the whole building may fall to pieces.

9) **Mind**, **prana** (breathing force, life force), and **semen** (**veerya**) are one. By controlling the mind, one can control the **prana** and semen. By controlling the **prana**, one can gain control over the mind and semen. By controlling the semen, one can gain control over the **mind** and **prana**. Mastery over any one of these brings control over the other two. **Mind**, **Prana**, and **Veerya** (**semen**) are under one connection or circuit (**sambandha**).

10) If **semen (veerya)** is controlled and if the energy used to create semen is made to flow upward into the brain by pure thoughts and practice of yogic postures, devotional services, etc., then the mind and **prana** are automatically controlled. This results in prodigious conservation of energy.

11) The mind is set in motion or rendered active by two things: the vibration of **prana** and the activation of subtle desires **(vasanas)**. When the mind is absorbed within itself, the **prana** is also restrained and then fixed. When the **prana** is fixed, the mind's inner absorption within itself increases. In *this* absorption, sexual energy now has a foundation for transformation.

12) When a man is excited by sexual passion, the **prana** is set into motion. The whole body obeys the dictates of the mind just as a soldier obeys the command of his commander. The vital air or **prana** moves the internal sap or semen. Hence, the semen gets put into motion.

13) If semen is lost via **ejaculatory orgasm**, **prana** gets unsteady and agitated, leading to disturbance in the cohesiveness of one's psycho-emotive structure. Mental processes also significantly change due to entrance into the refractory period where there is **negative relaxation**, sense of satisfaction, and overall reduction in consciousness.

14) The yogic traditions claim that the highest energy in the body is **ojas**. The **ojas** is powerful spiritual energy that is stored up in the brain and provides remarkable intellectual and spiritual strength. Great power of speech, language, and refinement in the quality of thoughts and emotions improve substantially as **ojas** is stored.

15) In each man, the **ojas** energy is stored to some extent or another and it can be considered that there are a multitude of forces at work that create **ojas**. The existence of **ojas** is a matter of transformation and not suppression or artificial control.

16) Multifaceted energies in the body (e.g. muscular energy, emotional energy, thought power, energy within desire, etc.) all becomes stored as **ojas** due to sex energy sublimation.

17) According to yogic traditions, sex energy is part of overall energy within the human body. The expression of sex energy in the form of sexual thoughts and desires, when diverted away from orgasmic experiences, creates openings in energy centers (**chakras**). This leads to storage of sex energy in the brain/mind as **ojas,** which is used for the benefit of the world due to sex energy not being funneled through the human ego. In most people, sex energy flows through the ego.

18) There exists a large amount of energy in all body fluids. Semen has the potency to create life. The conservation of sex energy, via semen sublimation, develops one's inner life and gives a "rebirth" to one's spiritual life. The significance of stopping of wastage of this great life force is realized by enlightened **yogis** (spiritual masters). The loss of this fluid is called the "little death" and it is from this "little death" that new life is created in the form of a child.

19) Each person's body is temporary, and remaining mostly focused on physical pleasures may not be the best use of the body. Excessive focus on physical pleasures leads to fear and suffering due to the wave-like nature of pleasure that cannot be sustained indefinitely. Limited pleasure can increase debt that must be paid later in life. The example of cigarette smoking is an excellent example of this debt. Pursuit of excessive pleasures increases one's debt — a debt that will be collected with interest at some point in one's life.

20) Real conservation of sexual fluids (i.e. **brahmacharya – celibacy**) starts with the purification of mental activity and careful attention to diet. Distinct types of food have different effects on metabolism, which affect the quality of emotional and cognitive (i.e. thinking process) functioning occurring within the mind. A vegetarian diet is recommended in this path. Even onions, garlic, and other spices, at times, can have aphrodisiac effects. It is also recommended by some spiritual teachers that one who is following the path of strict celibacy should cook one's own food, given that food carries considerable vibration of the preparer of the food.

21) Appreciation of the importance of diverting sex energy away from orgasmic pleasure must be strengthened by someone following the path of control. The continual diversion of sex energy away from frictional orgasm allows for this energy to be available for experiencing refined pleasures in life, such as music, literature, religion, scientific study, and spiritual awakening.

22) Clarity about using conserved sex energy for the benefit of others is also an integral part of the path of control. Controlled and conserved sex energy is used by **monks/sages/sadhus/mystics** for the benefit of humanity and their own spiritual advancement. They are extremely careful to not allow this energy to be spent by orgasmic experiences. Even if one is not a monk/sage, one who is interested in benefitting from sex energy conservation can use stored sex energy for society's benefit and **inner awakening**.

23) Awareness of suppression effects is the most critical inner exploration that one must perform while on the path of control. Suppression leads to a pendulum effect where one swings to indulgence, which causes further sex energy fragmentation. Many who are on the path of control are stuck in this problem of suppression and indulgence due to desire being controlled and not transformed.

24) Regular exercise, breath stabilization, and yogic postures are also an integral part of the sex energy sublimation using control of desire. These provide an adequate balance so that the energy within desire can **transmute** without the problems of suppression and indulgence.

25) Recognizing the division between the **controller and the controlled** is indispensable in preventing intra-psychic conflicts.

26) Establishing a relationship with God, if one is religiously inclined, can stabilize sexual energy, and **transmutation** can occur via prayers, contemplative meditations, and other religious practices.

27) Establishing a relationship with a higher power (i.e. higher energy) via sex sublimation is *absolutely necessary* in the path of control. This higher energy is necessary for sexual essences to flow upward rather than downward.

A relationship with God must transcend psychological projection of God. Direct contact with God requires sex energy to transmute via pure devotion. Emotions become purified and energy moves without friction when pure devotion flowers. -- Sachin J. Karnik

CHAPTER 5

MIND, SEX ENERGY& PSYCHOLOGICAL FRAGMENTATION

RELATIONSHIP BETWEEN THE MIND AND SEX ENERGY

There is, perhaps, no greater mystery in life than one's own mind. The "mind is the set of cognitive faculties that enables consciousness, perception, thinking, judgment, and memory. It is present in each human being.[1]" Each of us is conscious of our mind that produces a variety of thoughts, emotions, feelings, and desires. Figure 9 shown below depicts four interconnected aspects of what is known as the "mind" and also shows that sex energy exists within *each* aspect of it.

FIGURE 9
FOUR ASPECTS OF THE MIND & SEX ENERGY

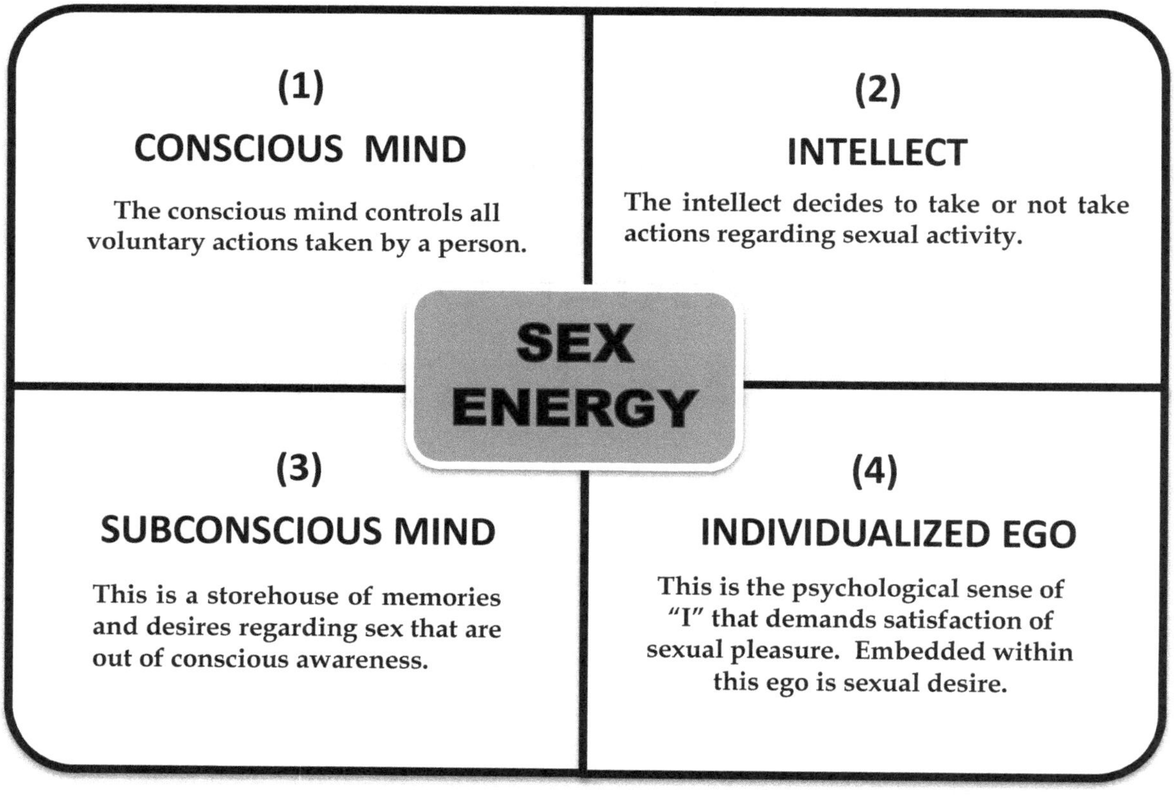

(1) CONSCIOUS MIND	(2) INTELLECT
The conscious mind controls all voluntary actions taken by a person.	The intellect decides to take or not take actions regarding sexual activity.
(3) SUBCONSCIOUS MIND	**(4) INDIVIDUALIZED EGO**
This is a storehouse of memories and desires regarding sex that are out of conscious awareness.	This is the psychological sense of "I" that demands satisfaction of sexual pleasure. Embedded within this ego is sexual desire.

SEX ENERGY (center)

The figure shown above has four boxes that all intersect with the "**sex energy**" box. Sex energy is one's "**root energy**" and is also known as "**Kundalini**." Kundalini is a **Sanskrit** term described in Eastern spiritual traditions as an internal spiritual energy that exists within one's physical body and mind. It is also known as "**shakti,**" which means power or corporeal energy that is responsible for the functioning of the entire body and all four functions of the mind as shown in figure 9. The **conscious mind** (box 1) is responsible for controlling all voluntary actions. These actions all use energy. For example, if a person walks one mile, energy is required to perform this activity. The energy required to do this exists within muscles, blood, bones, etc. The brain is the command center that sends impulses to the muscles to contract, and thus, moves the entire body. This entire process requires energy. This energy comes from food, and the energy within food is broken down, absorbed in the body, and stored in many different forms. There is considerable amount of energy transformed into sex energy which is stored in the brain, spinal cord, and generally present throughout the body. This energy is used in sexual stimulation where the experience of orgasmic pleasure uses vast amounts of this stored energy. **Kundalini** is sex energy that can be transmuted/transformed, as discussed earlier, into a refined form known as **ojas**. The awakening of **Kundalini** is synonymous with the expression "sex energy sublimation." If this great energy is sublimated, either with non-sexual meditation practices or using sex pleasure to move into sublimation as shown later in this book, then there is every possibility of purifying the subtle system within oneself and ultimately entering into a state of unblocked ecstasy and non-diluted joy. This purification leads to a state of connection with even greater powers within the universe and a possibility of direct connection with the spiritual dimension of reality. Such purification is non-fragmentation that occurs when there is adequate "inner awakening." This inner awakening is possible when there is recognition of major causes of sex energy fragmentation and one's personal desire to end this fragmentation. Figure 10 shows 14 major causes of sex energy fragmentation. Once this fragmentation has ended, a natural awakening of the **Kundalini** (root energy at the base of the spine) unblocks one's psychological system and takes one to a state of great joy, steadiness, and clarity. **Kundalini** itself is an instinctive or libidinal force that is mostly unconscious and exists as a great potentiality. The awakening of this **Kundalini** energy removes harmful patterns of negative emotion and bring great energy to one's neuropsychological system. This energy then can be used to accomplish great tasks for the betterment of oneself, one's family, and society in general. With great power comes great responsibility. Those who have awakened this **kundalini** use this energy to succeed in multiple aspects of one's life, ranging from financial success to spiritual progress.

This sex energy (**Kundalini**) gives energy to the conscious mind, the intellect, the subconscious mind, and the ego, as depicted in figure 9. To understand this with greater clarity, here are a few examples that illustrate how this sex energy is utilized by the four aspects of the mind:

1) The **conscious mind** controls all voluntary actions. The energy required to move the body, to contract muscles, to move bones, etc., is neuropsychological energy, muscular energy, and in a general sense, all physiological energy. This energy has its source ultimately from the sun. The sun's energy is transmitted into the food we eat, and our bodies break food into simpler

molecules. These molecules have energy that is then transformed ultimately into sex energy, which is the most refined form of the energy that is stored from food that has been consumed.

2) The **intellect** decides to take or not take actions regarding any action, including sexual activity. The decision-making ability within the human brain uses energy. Conserved sex energy (through pre-orgasmic conservation techniques or through natural sublimation) gives great power to the intellect. In most people, there is confusion about many decisions that must be made in life. The intellect that is infused with refined sex energy has increased capacity to think over multiple options, visualize pros and cons, and make decisions with a wide vision.

3) The **subconscious mind** is a storehouse of memories and desires that have been accumulating since birth. Past experiences of pleasure place pressure on the conscious mind to re-experience the same pleasure regarding sexual enjoyment. The subconscious mind operates in the background and is not in conscious awareness. During the dream state, the contents within the subconscious mind will emerge. The energy required to create the dream world is neuropsychological energy. If this energy in refined form (i.e. sex energy **transmutation**), is conserved, such conservation has the capacity to eventually take one into a state of restful sleep without excessive dreaming. Dreaming utilizes copious amounts of one's energy. If dreaming decreases, there is greater calmness in the mind due to the mind having enhanced energy. This energy is mostly fragmented and distorted in the dream state. Concentration of fragments occurs in the creation of the dream world. The creation of the dream world uses a great deal of energy that is wasted due to deep-seated conflicts and confusions that tear apart sex energy to create the dream world. Advanced meditators have the ability to "clean up" the dream state, resulting in the quality of dreams becoming positive, and eventually the amount of dreaming decreases substantially into a state known as "**yog nidra**." This is a state where all energy fragmentation effects have ended, and the dream state has been transformed into a deep restorative state.

4) The **individualized ego** is the psychological sense of "I" that demands satisfaction of sexual pleasure. Embedded within this ego is sexual desire. This "I" is one's psychological identity that uses great energy to satisfy desires. Desire is intimately associated with the "I" and the pressure of sexual desire demands relief where the "I" and the "impulses of desire" are essentially one. The ego works with the intellect, the conscious mind, and the subconscious mind to satisfy sexual desire. This satisfaction is experienced in the refractory period of the sexual response cycle.

The ego is the dividing factor in life. Desire and ego are intimately connected. Meditation allows one to see the difference between desire and ego, and this difference leads to inner freedom. In this freedom, sex energy is utilized by one's intelligence for fabulous growth in one's outward and inner life.

-- Sachin J. Karnik

PORNOGRAPHY & THE MIND

"The New York Times Magazine ran a cover story on May 18 called "Naked Capitalists: There's No Business Like Porn Business." Its thesis: Pornography is big business–with $10 billion to $14 billion in annual sales. The author, Frank Rich, suggests that pornography is bigger than any of the major league sports, perhaps bigger than Hollywood. Porn is "no longer a sideshow to the mainstream...it is the mainstream."[2]

Pornography is a growing business and a tremendous amount of money is spent on it, from $10 billion to $14 billion in annual sales, as stated above. When we look at such an enormous number, we can see that the vast numbers of individuals purchasing porn are essentially obtaining powerful neuropsychological stimulation that can produce potent sexual pleasure. In the previous section, we examined four aspects (or functions) of the mind that are intricately connected to the brain. The brain is truly the "largest" sex organ given that sexual desire and related neurological processes are occurring within it.

In an attempt to provide greater stimulation and satisfaction of sexual impulses, the advent of pornography (e.g. blue films, X-rated movies, etc.) has become a worldwide technological phenomenon since the invention of the VCR and DVD players. Now, with the internet, pornographic materials are readily available. There is no doubt that countless men and women throughout the world view pornographic materials as a means of sexual gratification. The question is: "Can pornography be used for psycho-spiritual development?" This may be a shocking question for many people, and those who are watching pornography may have never asked such a question. This question has immense importance, given that large numbers of people regularly watch pornography. Hence, is there a way to infuse meditation practices while watching pornography? Many people watch pornography as a means of experiencing quick and potent orgasmic pleasure. As discussed earlier, the mind/brain uses quite a bit of energy in the generation of a peak pleasurable experience. Ergo, the possibility of this energy being diverted via meditation is worthy of consideration. The amount of money, time, effort, and overall mental energy used in obtaining and viewing pornography is truly astounding. There is quite a bit of other energy used in the process as well. For example, money is energy because it has buying power. Purchasing pornographic materials is buying pleasure, escape, and a variety of other emotive and cognitive states.

Traditionally, most religions/spiritual paths have considered viewing pornography as a lustful act, sinful act, or at least, a non-spiritual act that takes one away from God or spirituality. As discussed earlier, a person on the "path of control" would probably take this viewpoint. If individuals are making spiritual progress on the "path of control" then that is well and good. There are individuals on the "path of control" who are trying to make progress toward sex sublimation, and they have quite a bit of difficulty at times.

Many such individuals secretly watch pornographic materials when "sexual tension" is heightening, and they lose their conserved sex energy via masturbation or sexual contact. The availability of instant pornography has great temptation for many who are trying to sublimate their sexual energy. In any case, watching porn can be a quick and easy way to have a personal simulative experience. Truly, the brain is the largest sex organ and watching porn allows the brain to generate orgasmic pleasure, on demand! The mystery of one's own mind, with regards to sexual processes, can be explored in multiple ways, including watching pornography *meditatively*, if one is so inclined.

Also, the amount of pleasure generated by watching pornography can be substantially higher than usual sexual connection between partners. According to neurobiological researchers, the amount of pleasure generated by pornography has significant effects on the brain. Internet pornography affects both the reward circuitry of the brain and the overall arousal process in the **reticular activation system**. This circuitry is highly complex and intricate that creates the experience of pleasure. The concept of reward, neurologically, refers to the experience generated by the release of neurotransmitters that modulate the experience of pleasure when neural connections change based on experiences inputted into the brain. Watching pornography strongly stimulates the reward circuitry in the ventral striatum. The level of activity in this area determines the degree to which various stimuli and self-pleasuring behavior create the experience of pleasure due to reward. Rewards come in multiple types, ranging from eating sweets to looking at erotic pictures, etc. These are known as **atavistic rewards**. These rewards refer to the reappearance in an individual of certain characteristics of our ancestors such as fascination with sexual stimulation.[3]

According to the theory of evolution, each human being is programmed to seek high calorie foods and find attractive mates due to the survival instinct. It should be noted that cocaine also activates the ventral striatum and creates an intense experience of euphoria. Watching pornography has the effect of retraining the brain. In the book "*The Brain That Changes Itself*," psychiatrist Norman Doidge explains:

"The men at their computers looking at porn ... had been seduced into pornographic training sessions that met all the conditions required for plastic change of brain maps. Since neurons that fire together wire together, these men got massive amounts of practice wiring these images into the pleasure centers of the brain, with the rapt attention necessary for plastic change. ... Each time they felt sexual excitement and had an orgasm when they masturbated, a 'spritz of **dopamine**', the reward neurotransmitter, consolidated the connections made in the brain during the sessions. Not only did the reward facilitate the behavior; it provoked none of the embarrassment they felt purchasing Playboy at a store. Here was a behavior with no 'punishment', only reward.

The content of what they found exciting changed as the Web sites introduced themes and scripts that altered their brains without their awareness. Because plasticity is competitive, the brain maps for new, exciting images increased at the expense of what had previously attracted them – the reason, I believe, they began to find their girlfriends less of a turn-on ... As for the patients who became involved in porn, most were able to go cold turkey once they understood the problem and how they were plastically reinforcing it. They found eventually that they were attracted once again to their mates."[4,5]

Pornography has the potentiality of hijacking primitive appetites and various biochemical mechanisms deeply imbedded as part of the neurobiology of the brain. Ancient neurological structures naturally pressure individuals toward behavior that evolution favors, which includes the pursuit of novel mates who bring the benefit of limiting inbreeding. Researchers have stated "porn addicts reported, that because of excessive use of sexually explicit materials, they had experienced diminished libido or erectile function, specifically in physical relationships with women, although not in relationship to the sexually explicit material."[6,7]

When watching pornography, arousal is not necessarily slow, relaxed, and built-up as in usual sexual contact. There is a jump to direct high energy orgasmic experience in the mind of the one watching explicit images. There is also a considerable amount of novelty regarding the content of internet pornography. There are, of course, individuals addicted to pornography and those who enjoy it *without* becoming addicted. Key features of any addiction are as follows: difficulty in stopping the activity when the appetite for it increases; increased habituation of the activity where there is need for more and more stimulation; and personal problems (i.e. social, familial, financial, etc.) that are caused by the activity. Given that most current pornography now comes in high resolution, there is even greater conditioning in the mind for that type of stimulation, which is very far removed from actual sexual activity with real people. The mind becomes increasingly conditioned to high definition pornography. *The mixture of meditation into watching sexual acts while one is masturbating may open a doorway into greater awareness of one's own sexual processes.* These techniques are discussed in chapter 7.

The pursuit of beautiful and attractive women, and the idealization of desirable women in cinema, print ads, etc.) create unrealistic sexual expectations in actual relationships. Porn creates even greater unrealistic physical form expectations and performance expectations. The question becomes, how can strong sexual excitation occur when one's partner (married, etc.) is NOT as physically attractive as a fantasized form or porn actor/actress? To maintain novelty with the same partner is possible through meditative sexual practices. This requires the "desire-connection" to remain active via ending in energy and not in loss of desire. To make that happen, steady yet expanding mini-orgasms are required to create deep satisfaction (satiety), keep desire active, and reengage in sexual stimulation. Sexual desire remains active due to avoiding the **point-of-no-return**. This avoidance is done very meditatively and intelligently due to clear inner recognition and realization that going to the **point-of-no-return** actually breaks contact between male/female energies and has many possible consequences, such as reduction of energy, loss of desire, and breakage of emotional connectivity between partners.

WHAT IS PSYCHOLOGICAL FRAGMENTATION?

Figure 10 depicts 14 major causes of sex energy fragmentation. Before examining these areas in detail, the meaning of "**fragmentation**" needs to be understood clearly. "**Fragmentation**" refers to the fact that most people's lives are split apart psychologically, when various fragmented pieces conflict with each other. Here are several examples of psychological fragmentation:

a) Any given person plays distinct roles in various parts of his/her life. These parts include home life, office life, political life, sexual life, etc. Although it is necessary to play separate roles in various settings, the mind of most human beings has become internally conflicted. For example, a man has a strong relationship with his wife, yet his sexual desires are pressuring him to seek other relationships for sexual gratification.

b) Frustrations at work causes a mother to come home and yell at her children for no apparent reason. This frustration is carried over due to the mother being internally fragmented (i.e. distressed, overwhelmed, etc.) by her situation at work. Her relationship with her significant other may be imbalanced, and this has resulted in her not being sexually satisfied.

c) A 25-year-old man has a girlfriend and is interested in developing a deeper emotional relationship with her. She is also interested in a deeper relationship, yet she feels sexually dissatisfied due to her partner not being able to sexually satisfy her to the point of experiencing 4 powerful orgasms. She barely experiences one orgasm while her partner has already ejaculated and entered into a refractory period.

d) An individual has taken a vow of celibacy as part of his/her spiritual path. The path of celibacy has been difficult, and the individual reverts to watching pornography excessively and satisfies sexual desires via masturbation. After sexual impulses are satisfied, there is a profound sense of guilt, shame, and a deep sense of failure on the spiritual path. The individual reverts to spiritual practices and refrains from masturbating for about 1 month. After that time, sexual desire and pressure increase to the point that reversion back to pornography seems inevitable. There is a true war going on inside the mind of this person where sexual energy is torn apart by trying to control powerful sexual impulses on one hand and then indulging with great force on the other hand. This is a pendulum effect that creates and enhances psychological division and energy fragmentation.

> ***Fragmentation is the main problem within the mind. Different pieces of thoughts, emotions, memories, and desires exist as interrelated and interconnected fragments that are internally contradictory. This contradiction tears apart sex energy. -- Sachin J. Karnik***

MAJOR CAUSES OF SEX-ENERGY FRAGMENTATION

There are at least 14 major causes of psychological fragmentation as depicted in figure 10. Described below is a description of each cause and how it fragments sex energy:

1) *Unsatisfied Sexual Desire*
   Desire, by definition, is the lack of satisfaction or fulfillment. When sexual desire remains unfulfilled or is not satisfied the way one wants it satisfied, then frustration ensues, resulting in emotional energy being torn apart. **Emotional energy** is intricately tied to the fountain-like flow of desires within oneself. Emotional energy is one aspect of one's full sex energy (**Kundalini**). If there are emotional frustrations due to the constant presence of unfulfilled desire, then these frustrations fragment energy. Fragmented energy gets further split due to increased focus on the lack of emotional satisfaction.

2) *Difficulty in Attracting the Opposite Sex*
   Many individuals have difficulty in attracting the opposite sex of one's choice. This can cause deep internal dissatisfaction as well as a sense of low self-esteem. These negative emotional states can further fragment energy and cause a great deal of self-criticism and other inner problems.

3) *Hyper-sexuality*
   Some people have frequent or sudden increases of libido. Sometimes this is also known as **nymphomania**. This can occur for a variety of reasons, and there are some people with mental health issues that have these problems. In a more generic sense, hyper-sexuality is a type of over stimulation within the brain that causes sex energy to fragment and deeper fixation with sexual stimulation can occur. This deeper fixation with sexual stimulation leads to one's mind pursuing orgasmic pleasures to the point of causing damage to the brain's natural pleasure system.

4) *Unfulfilled Fantasies about Sexual Situations*
   Fantasy is a big part of sexual stimulation. Fantasy is part of one's mental framework in sexual stimulation. **Sexual fantasy** has mental images of an erotic nature that can possibly lead to sexual arousal. There are explicitly erotic feelings that are accompanied by changes in the physical body that occur as a result of arousal. The fantasy creation process occurs within the mind itself. The mind yearns for a type of stimulation aiming to experience sexual arousal leading to orgasm. When fantasies are not fulfilled or partially fulfilled, this creates sex energy fragmentation, leading to further attempt to reach a fully satisfied state.

5) *Negative Perceptions of One's Sexual Appeal*
   Self-image, **self-worth**, and **self-esteem** are all related and contained in one's perception of one's own sexual appeal. When there is negative self-perception, an inner sense of "not being OK with oneself" occurs, which causes disturbances within one's identity structure leading to fragmentation of energy.

6) *Low Self-Esteem*
   Self-esteem is an emotional evaluation of one's own perception of oneself. Low levels of self-esteem can result in decrease of overall energy. Decrease in energy can also lead to low self-esteem. This decrease in energy can lead to possible damage to energy levels. Diminutions in overall energy can affect sexual energy levels and not allow healthy functioning of sexual processes. Self-esteem is related to academic achievement, satisfaction in marriage, and accomplishment of many other goals in life. The energy fragmentation effects of low self-esteem can lead to sex energy not flowing properly. When energy fragmentation stops, there is great cohesion of self-worth, self-respect, and self-integrity.

7) *Homeostatic Imbalances*
   Imbalances in one's physical and mental health can cause considerable destruction of sexual energy. **Homeostasis** refers to a state of overall physical and neuropsychological balance that the body/mind is constantly trying to maintain.

8) *Problems in One's Spiritual Path*
   Difficulties in one's religious/spiritual path can cause frustration and lead to sexual energy being disturbed. These disturbances in one's spiritual path can lead to self-imposed suppression or severe indulgence. The pendulum effect between suppression and indulgence is a fundamental problem for many on a religious or spiritual path. The pulling back and forth of sexual energy via indulgence and suppression fragments it, and can cause one to fall away from one's chosen religious/spiritual path.

9) *Novelty Seeking in Sexual Stimulation to The Point of Saturation*
   Novelty in sexual simulation occurs due to a sense of repetition of the same type(s) of stimulation. The problem of repetition is serious because excessive pursuit of novelty leads to saturation. Saturation is the state where further desire for stimulation is not present or there is excessive boredom despite experiencing a wide range of novel sexual situations. The fragmentation effect is solidified when this occurs and has the potential of damaging desire for sexual stimulation.

10) *Problems with Significant Other*

Conflicts in relationships can cause considerable disturbances within one's energy structure. Relationships can become toxic due to increased conflicts and misunderstandings. Disturbances in intimacy can break **inner cords** of healthy attachment that affect the flow of emotions and overall heath. Any time one choses to enter a sexual relationship with another person, an "energy cord" is created with the person. This energy cord is an energy connection between partners and disturbances in this connection causes sex energy to fragment. Sexual connection with another person has depth when energy is activated and connected during the formation of the experience of pleasure. Sharing of intimate energy has profound effects on the body and mind. Various impressions (**samskaras**) are formed in the mind of the person having intimate contact because there is an exchange of energies. The fragmentation effect caused by imbalance within intimacy needs to be cleared physically and emotionally. Combining meditation with intimacy is a path for clearing energy imbalances. If one is involved in multiple relationships, then energy transference can be even more complex. Again, meditation is the key in clearing up disturbances. Energy can be negative or positive, based on the vibration of one's partner and one's own vibration. It is possible for one's partner's thoughts, feelings, unresolved emotions, and other disturbances to become intertwined with one's psychological life. If this intertwining has negativity within it, it can cause greater disintegration of psychological energy. The use of alcohol or other drugs with sexual stimulation will further lower positive energy and possibly open the door into lower levels of consciousness. This is especially true if the brain is hyper stimulated by illicit drugs. The quality of sexual energy can get polluted by the mixture of alcohol and/or other illicit substances. Rather than sexual energy getting revitalized naturally, it gets hyper-stimulated by certain drugs and can cause more damage. As a result, problems with one's significant other can possibly worsen if alcohol and/or other drugs are used excessively with sexual stimulation.

11) *Negative Memories about Past Sexual Experiences*

If there are negative memories about past sexual experiences, then those memories will further fragment sexual energy. This occurs when one is trying to engage in sexual activity due to negative memories contaminating sexual stimulation.

12) *Alcohol, Tobacco, Other Drugs, and Gambling (ATOD & G)*

The use of substances such as alcohol, tobacco, and other drugs (e.g. heroin, cocaine, etc.) and/or gambling will further fragment the natural flow of sexual energy. These substances can, at times, temporarily increase or decrease sexual desires and eventually lead to degradation of sexual energy due to excessive stimulation of the reward circuitry in the brain.

13) *Mental Health Problems*

Problems with depression, anxiety, bipolar disorder, etc., can all fragment natural sexual energy. For example, chronic depression can affect **libido**, and this causes sex energy to fragment. Mental health problems, in general, can affect sexual desire, cause difficulty in reaching orgasm, erection difficulty in men, among other problems.

14) *Negative or Painful Emotions*

Negative emotions or current/past painful emotions will definitely fragment sexual energy. Negative emotions utilize large amounts of energy that should be available for normal activities in life, including the generation of sexual pleasure. Here is a list of negative emotions and mental qualities that can easily fragment sexual energy and degrade it further:

Abusive – Controlling – Aggressive – Cowardly – Greedy – Angry – Critical – Grieving –Annoyed
Cruel – Hatred – Antagonistic – Defeated – Hopeless – Anxious – Deluded – Ignorant – Arrogant
Demanding – Impatient – Ashamed – Dependent – Impoverished – Belligerent – Depressed
Impulsive - Bitter - Desperate - Indifferent Bored - Destitute - Inert - Broken-down - Destructive
Insecure - Bullied - Detached - Insensitive - Chaotic - Disconnected - Irresponsible - Cold
Discouraged - Irritated - Commanding - Disgusted - Isolated - Competitive - Dominated - Jealous
Complaining - Dominating - Judged - Conceited - Egocentric - Judgmental - Condemned
Egotistical -Lazy – Conflicted – Envious – Lonely - Confused - Erratic - Lost - Conservative
Frightened - Mad - Controlled - Frustrated - Manipulated - Manipulative - Ridiculous - Unhappy
Miserable - Righteous - Unresponsive - Moody - Ruthless - Untrusting - Moral - Sad – Vain
Negative – Sadistic - Vengeance - Secretive - Vicious - Obsessed - Self condemning – Victimized
Panicked - Self-defeating - Violent - Paranoid - Self-destructive - Wise – Passive - Self-hatred
Perfectionist - Self-obsessed - Pitiful - Self-pity - Poor - Self-sabotaging – Possessive - Selfish
Preoccupied - Shamed - Procrastination - Shut down - Punished - Shy – Punishing - Sorry
Rage – Stricken - Reactionary - Strung out - Reclusive - Stubborn – Rejected – Superior
Repressed – Tantrums – Resentful – Timid – Resigned – Unconcerned – Responsible
Unforgiving

Adequate mixture of meditation with sexual stimulation can transform negative emotions and negative mental stages into positive rejuvenation of energy.

-- Sachin J. Karnik

FIGURE 10

MAJOR CAUSES OF SEX ENERGY FRAGMENTATION

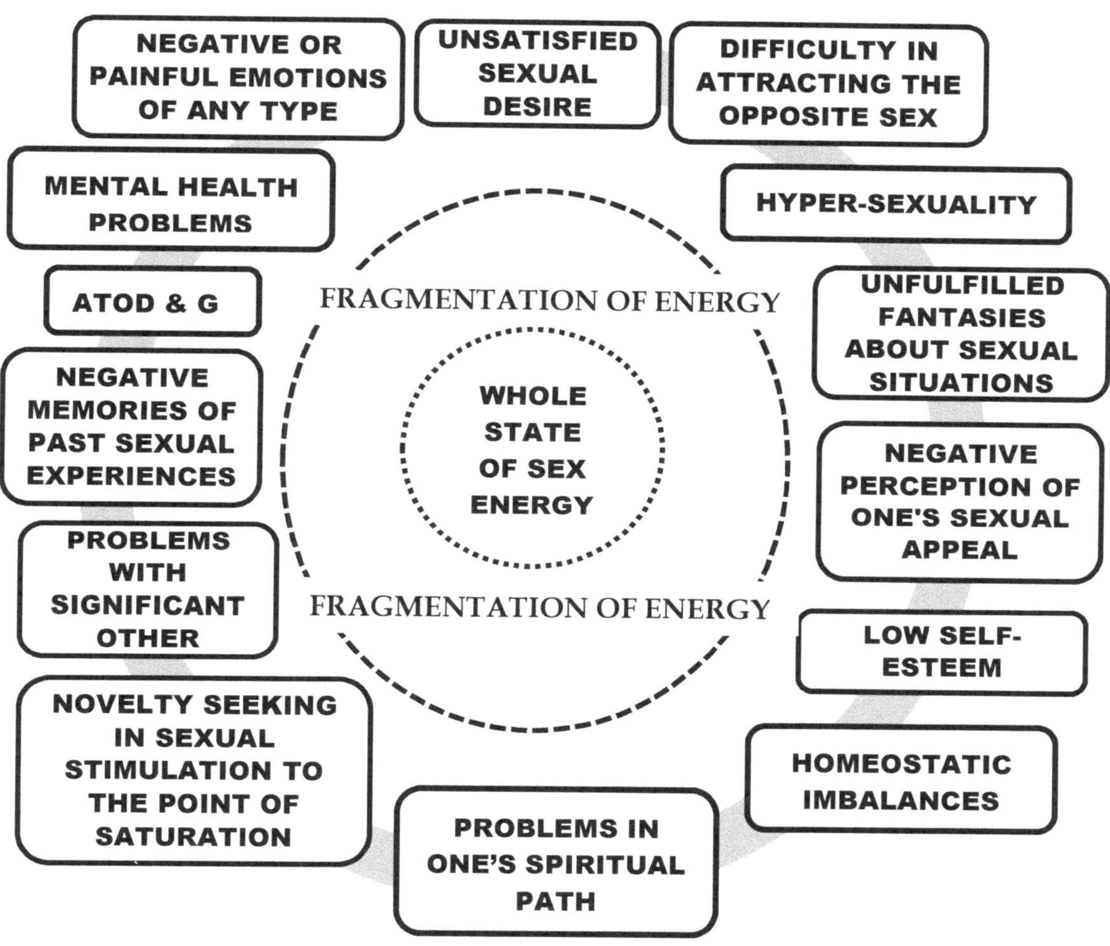

The "whole state" of sex energy has nearly unlimited capacity to open fantastic possibilities in one's life. When sex energy is no longer fragmented, it becomes sacred energy.

-- Sachin J. Karnik

CHAPTER 6

MEDITATION & SEX ENERGY TRANSMUTATION

COMBINING MEDITATION & PLEASURE: FUSION OF SEX ENERGY

So far, the nature of sex energy fragmentation has been examined. This fragmentation effect is predominant in most people's minds and creates many difficulties that do not allow for true inner satisfaction where copious energy becomes available for enjoying life to its fullest. In this chapter, we will explore together the central idea of "fusion" of male and female energies. This internal fusion aims to eliminate psychological fragmentation and brings about a state of inner wholeness. Such inner wholeness is a state of pure joy, happiness, and balance where internal blocks, tensions, and contradictions have come to an end. Foundational understanding of the principles of inner fusion of male and female sex energies is provided in this chapter. Such a foundation is necessary to understand the purpose behind various practices shown in chapter 7. These practices utilize sexual pleasure as a means of progressing toward a state of ecstasy and ultimately, toward a state of pure joy (**ananda**).

As stated before, sex energy is fragmented in most individuals. It is possible to fuse broken energy back into a whole state *without* the denial of pleasure. The ancient tradition of **tantra** advocates for the mixture of meditation in the pleasures of life, especially sexual pleasure. Some basic understanding of the principles of **tantra** is necessary to set the foundation for understanding chapter 7, which discusses the power of pre-orgasmic sex energy transmutation. So, what is **tantra**? **Tantra** is an ancient Asian meditation practice that uses sexual energies for embracing sensual pleasures and utilizes these sensual pleasures for the purpose of psycho-spiritual awakening. One definition of **tantra**, according to David Gordon White, is:

"**Tantra** is that Asian body of beliefs and practices which, working from the principle that the universe we experience is nothing other than the concrete manifestation of the divine energy of the Godhead that creates and maintains that universe, seeks to ritually appropriate and channel that energy, within the human microcosm, in creative and emancipatory ways.[1]"

Meditation is a direct way of transmuting sex energy. The principles of **tantra** that advocate for the infusion of meditation into sexual stimulation are as follows:

1) Meditation practices allow for accessing and getting directly in touch with one's intrinsic sexual energy.
2) Infusion of meditation into deep intimacy allows for the weaving together of fragmented thoughts, emotions, and energies. This "weaving together" is the essential meaning of **tantra**. Integration at this level allows for true connection between partners for mindful sexual practices.

3) Meditative awareness of the nature of pleasure generated in the sexual act allows for greater time to be spent in foreplay. Also, while engaging in intercourse, there is a possibility of greater inner union between couples due to enhanced sensitivity.
4) The infusion of meditation into feelings of sensuality can allow one to move into sexual stimulation *slowly*, resulting in increased awareness of the nature of pleasure. This increases awareness of one's body overall, erogenous zones in one's body, and the importance of healthy connection with one's partner.
5) The release of creative energy (**shakti**) that is lying dormant within each person is a major goal of combining pleasure and meditation together. Meditation practices, such as deep breathing, mindful awareness, mantra meditation, etc., can all be mixed with the activation of sexual pleasure. This creative energy is only minimally active in most people, and the infusion of meditation with energy activation in sexual stimulation will allow greater energy to be released.
6) The practice of meditation can lead to awareness of the existence of spiritual energy nerves known as "**nadis**." These have spiritual energy within them and the energy existing in these spiritual nerves manifests itself in the mind and the body, resulting in the interaction between the energy extracted from food and the energy existing in spiritual nerves. The existence of **nadis** cannot be proven scientifically, because they can *only* be perceived in deep meditation. Also, there are major energy plexuses called "**chakras,**" and these can also be perceived *only* in deep meditation. Advanced meditators describe the chakras as spinning vortices that are responsible for the creation of the experiences for the **soul** in the waking and dream state. Again, there is spiritual energy (**Kundalini**) that flows through the **chakras**. In most people, this energy is mostly blocked due to negative emotional states, negative thinking, worries about the future, and being trapped in the over analysis of past events in one's life. (See upcoming section on "**Psychological Time**.)
7) There is *only one energy* that assumes many forms. Mastery over the movement of energy occurs when one enters into a state of observation of the movement of energy. In such mastery, use of energy can take place in ways that are extremely mindful. The abuse and misuse of energy is responsible for considerable human suffering. Hence, an awakened intelligence is required to stop the abuse and misuse of energy.

The tradition of **tantra** (i.e. the infusion of meditation into pleasures of life) has been greatly misunderstood and misapplied over thousands of years. When there is positive feeling and good intention in pleasure activation, there can exist increased integration and overall psychological wellbeing. The principles of meditation propose certain ideas that are worthy of careful consideration. One major idea is that we are all **human microcosms**. (The **Sanskrit** term for the human microcosm is **pinda** and the macrocosm is the **Brahmanda**). Each of us is a part of the universe that we perceive through our senses. Therefore, each of us is an individual expression of the entire cosmos. This may seem highly esoteric and mystical. Nonetheless, there are some basic comparisons that highlight each human being as a miniaturized universe. The comparisons are shown in table 1 on the next page.

TABLE: 1
COMPARISON BETWEEN CONTENTS OF THE UNIVERSE AND THE HUMAN BODY

THE UNIVERSE ⟷	THE HUMAN BODY
The universe contains the five great elements (Physical Matter, Water, Chemical Reactions, Air, and Space)	The same five great elements are in our physical body, only in miniaturized form.
The universe contains an infinite amount of energy	The human body and mind are a miniaturized manifestation of this infinite energy. It is this infinite energy that is known as "**prana**" or sex energy.
Cosmic Intelligence	Human beings have the biggest brain among all the animals and hence, the greatest intelligence. This mental power is constantly linked to cosmic intelligence. Once we enter into a state of wholeness (i.e. non-fragmentation), a doorway opens into the infinite cosmic intelligence.
The cosmos known through science is a partial vision of what actually exists.	Deep meditation allows for an internal doorway to open up so that the entire cosmos can be seen. To open this doorway, great energy is required, and sublimated sex energy creates a foundation for the doorway to open.
The cosmos contains innumerable galaxies and star systems, as known through our study of science.	Each human being contains seven major spiritual centers (chakras) that are connecting points to the entire universe. Beyond the 7th chakra exists the infinite spiritual reality, which is beyond the cosmos. This can only be accessed through profound meditation.
There is great beauty in the universe. Each planet, each star, and each galaxy are extraordinary and a miracle of creation.	Each human being is a miracle of creation. Each human being is created as a part of the universe and has infinite beauty within. The beauty and sense of unending awe when we gaze into the night sky, see a sun rise, see the full moon, etc., *is a reflection* of our inner beauty. The beauty is in us, it is because of us, and it *is* us.

Anyone contemplating on the ideas presented in the table above, would be filled with a sense of wonder and curiosity as to what actually exists within oneself. To gain access to deeper realities within oneself that connect with the cosmos and trans-cosmic realities, it is absolutely necessary for the mind (i.e. thoughts, emotions, memories, desires, etc.) to awaken to a *state* of complete harmony and stability. This is perhaps the greatest challenge for humanity today. Due to great scientific advances, our lives have become easier and more comfortable. Nevertheless, humanity is still in its psychological infancy with endless conflicts at all levels within society. Figure 11 below illustrates that conflicts exist at all levels of society within which humanity is imprisoned.

FIGURE 11
THE PRISON OF HUMAN CONFLICTS

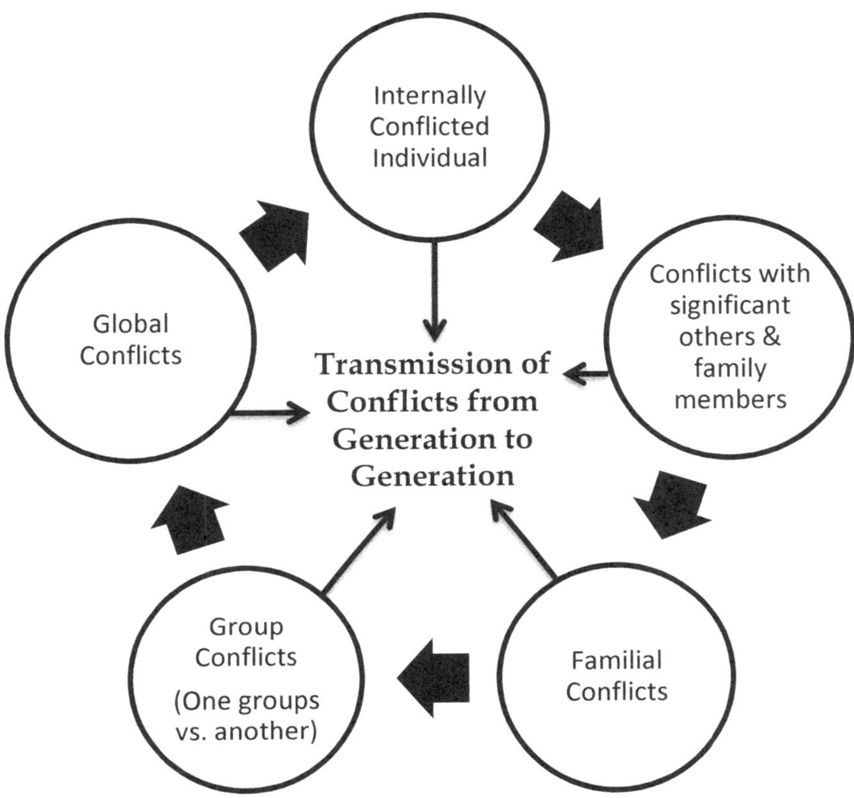

The central question that needs consideration is as follows: "How can a person come out of psychological conflicts and enter into wholeness?" In examining the figure above, we can see that humanity is stuck in the prison of conflict, because conflicts of all types are transmitted to the next generation. This transmission occurs via conditioning processes within the human brain/mind due to an individual's identity being formed with "conflict" as the status quo. This status quo has resulted in thousands of recorded wars in human history and in battles that continue in people's personal lives, in relationships, and within families.

Past human conflicts between racial, religious, and political groups are transmitted from one generation to another. This transmission process has imprisoned humanity in conflict at multiple levels. The author would like to emphasize that disagreement can be healthy if approached with the right spirit. Dislike, hatred, and ultimately violence, due to disagreement have poisoned the human mind. This poison can be eliminated from the root level in society if individuals learn how to access the fountain of pure joy that exists within. The creation of this access point is possible through harnessing sexual energy, either through practices shown in chapter 4 or practices that will be presented in chapter 7. The practices in chapter 7 *embrace* sexual pleasure as a means of creating an access point into the fountain of absolute joy. It is the author's contention that as harnessing of sexual energy become solidified, various fragments of emotions, thoughts, memories, desires, hopes, likes, dislikes, etc. all combine together and merge into each other, opening a gateway into the fountain of pure joy that exists within each of us. As we discussed earlier, the word, "**tantra**", means "weaving together" the various split parts within our personality. When sex energy begins to flow within one's psycho-physical system without fragmentation, then a natural weaving occurs within oneself. The state of **transformation/transmutation** that occurs after weaving together all fragmented pieces is depicted in figure 12 shown below:

FIGURE 12

SEX ENERGY TRANSMUTATION INTO PURE JOY

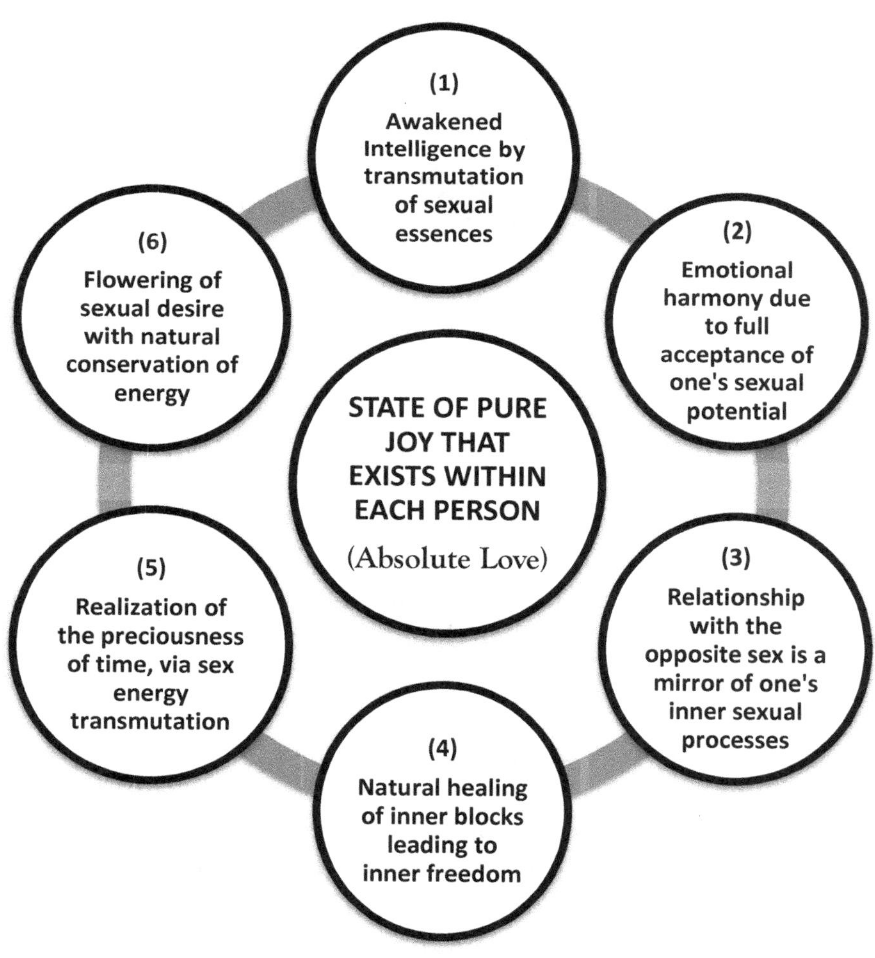

Sex energy **transmutation** can create an adequate psychological foundation that leads to **transformation** as shown in each of the six areas in figure 12. In considering each of these areas, the goals of **tantra** can lead to the ultimate goal of entering into and remaining in a state of pure joy. One's sexual energy is one's own raw power that can be harnessed without denying pleasure to create a gateway into a state of absolute joy. The advantages in performing the practices of **tantra** (e.g. pre-orgasmic sex, sacred sexuality, meditative sex, tantric sex, **karezza**, etc.) are: embracing pleasure rather than fighting with pleasure and using pleasure for greater purposes (i.e. deepening the bonds between couples; facilitating energy **transmutation**; and ultimately, entering into a state of pure, non-fragmented joy). These advantages are shown below in connection to the six results of sex energy **transmutation** (e.g. circles 1 to 6 in figure 12):

Advantage #1: *Expansion of love, resulting in personal and interpersonal emotional harmony (see circle #2 in figure 12).* This is due to the acceptance of sexual pleasure as a very natural aspect of one's being. This acceptance creates the foundation for using sexual processes and embraces sexual pleasures to discover within the fountain of absolute joy (**ananda**).

Advantage #2: *Physical and mental health rejuvenation and renewal, resulting in the natural healing of inner blocks (see circle #4 in figure 12).* The practices explained in chapter 7 place significant importance on cultivating awareness of one's breath with an emphasis on taking deeper breaths to nourish the physical body and mind.

Advantage #3: *Mixing meditation with sexuality can remove imbalances in relationships between partners.* Imbalances exist in intimate relationships. Mindfully slowing down sexual stimulation can gradually reduce emotional friction between partners. Sensitivity in an intimate relationship is an essential part of growth within the relationship.

Advantage #4: *Mixing meditation with sexual stimulation increases the possibility of rejuvenating health.* Rejuvenation refers to restoration back to an original or new state with new vigor and energy. Sexual stimulation releases considerable energy from the brain and many organs within the body. This energy, if harnessed properly, may have very good health benefits. Conserved energy can be used to strengthen the physical body, strengthen intellectual activities, bring balance to emotions, and eventually take the practitioner of meditative sexuality to a state of non-contradictory desire.

> ***Excellent physical and mental health requires energy to be used without a conflict between the mind and the body. This conflict can dissolve by mixing meditation with sexual stimulation, allowing energy to transmute.***
> ***-- Sachin J. Karnik***

Advantage #5: *Reduction of mental health problems such as anxiety and depression, along with improvements in self-esteem, confidence levels, and self-image are possible if the right types of meditation are mixed with sexual stimulation.*
(Warning: If you have mental health or addiction problems, please consult with your doctor, psychiatrist, or psychotherapist before attempting any practices shown in this book. There is no guarantee that mixing meditation with sexual stimulation will definitely reduce mental health or addiction problems. Practices of the mixture of meditation and sexual stimulation performed by individuals with mental health/addiction problems, should be done under the guidance of a trained professional.) Many common problems of depression, anxiety, etc., are generally mood problems or problems in emotional regulation. It is possible to activate and use *natural pleasure* that already exists within oneself in dormant form and use it for overall wellbeing. Notice that the author is emphasizing the "use of natural pleasure" for the benefit of the mind rather than the mind generating high levels of pleasure artificially via drugs, alcohol, gambling, hyper-sexuality, etc. The unlocking of natural pleasure is akin to unlocking a hidden treasure within oneself. This "hidden treasure" is unlocked meditatively, and therefore, the power of slowly unlocking it opens subtle layers that are mostly unknown to individuals.

Advantage #6: *Men can feel more empowered in sexual relationships given that many men struggle with premature ejaculation or they are highly focused on their own pleasure, which leads to inadequate sensitivity to their female partner's level of satisfaction.* Mixture of meditation with sexual stimulation can bring about long periods of intimate connection where true intimacy begins to develop. Intimacy can be expressed and experienced as: "INTO ME, YOU SEE, IS INTIMACY." Such deep connection also allows for female partners to experience multiple orgasms, while the male partner remains, meditatively, in pre-orgasmic stimulation. Various techniques for this type of pre-orgasmic meditation are described in chapter 7.

Advantage #7: *Mixing meditation with sensual and sexual stimulation can provide a foundation for opening deeper and richer dimensions in life.* Spiritual development can occur due to transformative processes taking place when meditation is carefully mixed with pleasure. The richness of life, via senses being fully active, can be experienced without being at war with pleasure. Being at war with sexual pleasure can produce many psychological problems. By the same token, pursuit of sexual pleasure to the point of hyper-sexuality may also be damaging to the mind/brain due to energy being destroyed that could have been available for the flowering of one's life in multiple directions.

> ***True intimacy is beyond linguistic expressions. Pure intimacy transmutes the ego's energy into love energy.***
> ***-- Sachin J. Karnik***

Advantage #8: *Sexual pleasure enhancement can occur via increased ejaculatory control in men where diversion of sexual energies can happen due to increased awareness of the movement of orgasmic power.* Increased awareness of the nature of orgasm can provide men a deeper personal connection with their own sexual response cycle. This increased personal connection expands awareness of the awakened inner female energy. This awakening is experienced in the form of orgasmic pleasure and can increase inner fusion of energies.

Advantage #9: *When mindful meditation is mixed with sexual stimulation, there is a strong possibility of enhanced connection in multiple areas within one's life.* **Transmutation** is the **transformation** via reconnection of broken energies into wholeness that opens the door for increased sensitivity and love for all of creation. Hence, enhanced connection without fragmentary and hyper-focused direction, allows for actual love within one's heart to open and connect with all of reality. There is increasing inner freedom in such a state of living where joy abides naturally, and the use of one's energy becomes very positive, impacting one's inner and outer world.

In most of us, our thoughts, emotions, actions, energies, and feelings are usually split apart and fragmented in many ways, as we saw in Chapter 5. This fragmentation causes internal conflicts, and thus, conflicts occur with others. The ultimate purpose of *any spiritual practice* is to discover a state of complete "wholeness." Wholeness is the goal of practices shown in chapter 7. Using sexual energies for the purpose of unlocking refined and enhanced bliss (i.e. moving from erotic to ecstatic states) within ourselves and ultimately, for the purpose of enlightenment, is certainly possible. If one's goal is to have a joy-filled life, then inner integration of sexual energies is necessary.

SYMBOLS OF MALE & FEMALE FUSION

In various Eastern traditions, there are several symbols that express the notion that the female exists in the male and that the male exists in the female. This is call the **Shiva Lingam** in India. This symbol represents the *inner fusion* of male and female energies. The erected upward form is a representation of the upward flow of sex energy. Also, it represents an erected penis that is joined with the female sex organ. This symbolic representation is indicative of inner fusion of sexual essences that are transmuted into divine light. Hence, the black color is representative of raw sexual desire and the white lines are representative of transmutation of raw energy into refined energy that can be experienced as divine light in deep meditation. The **Shiva Lingam** represents both male and female, as well as the cosmic egg from which all creation emerged. This symbol is an abstract or aniconic representation of the indivisible two-in-oneness of male and female inner sexual processes. All life originates from sexual energy and the Lingam represents the sublimation and transformation of this energy, inwardly.

SHIVA LINGAM

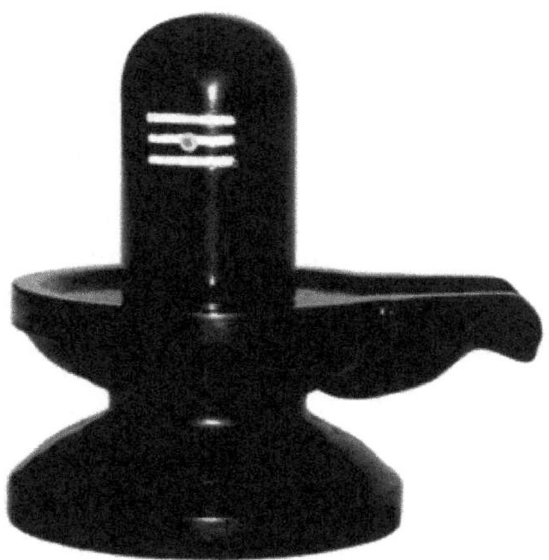

In Chinese philosophy, yin and yang, describe how seemingly opposite or contrary forces may actually be complementary, interconnected, and interdependent in the natural world, and how they may give rise to each other as they interrelate to one another.

The Chinese tradition has a very familiar symbol of the **Yin/Yang circle**. (See below).

YIN/YANG CIRCLE

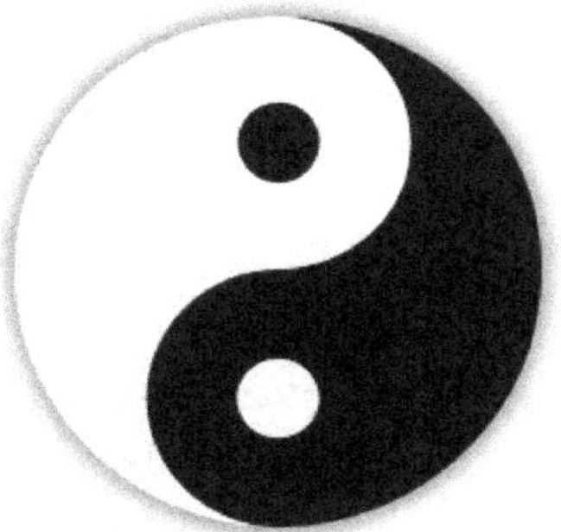

This symbol represents perfect and harmonic balance between male and female energies. Duality exists in life and can readily be seen. The **Yin** and **Yang** are considered to be part of *oneness* that is also likened with the **Tao**. The image shown above can be interpreted as follows: the white circle represents female energy; the black circle represents male energy and the two smaller circles represent the presence of male energy in the female and the female energy in the male. Philosophically, this is known as dualistic monism or dialectical monism where yin and yang are complementary rather than opposing processes/forces forming an intra-psychic energetic system that is the whole. Integration of opposing forces is the goal in **Taoist sexual practices**. These Taoist practices also have the same principle of combining meditation with sexual stimulation.

The usual discharge of orgasmic energy via orgasms is considered as a release of life-force power that occurs in the creation of the experience of pleasure. Orgasm is considered in many Eastern traditions to be a temporary fusion of polar energies that give a glimpse of a non-dual state. This glimpse of oneness can provide the foundation to experience a deeper oneness that is beyond concentrated orgasm. The inward flow of this energy is encouraged in Taoist sexual practices where there is reprocessing and greater qualitative enhancement of such energy. Considerable emphasis is also placed on staying in **valley orgasms** (or what the author has termed as, the "**mini-orgasmic sex energy current**") which allows for sexual desire to remain intact rather than being extinguished. The meditative cultivation of **valley orgasms** is possible when there is considerable slowing down of simulative processes. These **valley orgasms** (i.e. mini-orgasms) allow for greater energy release and deeper inner fusion of the **yin** and **yang** where energy is not lost but rejuvenates itself. When meditation is infused with simulative processes, it can provide a proper mental foundation for harnessing sex energy and cultivating it for other purposes that can have wonderful benefits in many areas of one's life. If the refractory period is avoided for extended periods of time, natural rejuvenation is possible and deeper realms of pleasure may open within oneself.

INNER RESEARCH

Avoidance of the refractory period requires an inner journey to take place. Inner research is required for progress toward greater inward cohesion of energy. Carl Jung said the following:

"Your vision will become clear only when you can look into your own heart. Who looks outside, dreams; who looks inside, awakens[2]." – Carl Jung

As the inward journey starts, one will find that creation of resistance of sexual pleasure may strengthen the demand for indulgence. This truth must be observed directly within oneself via silent meditation. Silent meditation is sitting alone and observing the polarity of the mind. Looking into one's own heart, as stated by Carl Jung in the quote above, requires brutal honesty where one clearly perceives without any inner disturbance. Realization of the existence of "inner disturbance" is a huge step in anyone's life. Most people simply live through their inner disturbances and have accepted them to be "just part of life." The "fusion of sex energy" where male and female aspects are intertwined creates a natural state of "non-disturbance." Disturbances present in daily life will begin to diminish significantly as this fusion process takes hold. Within each male there is female energy and within each female there is the need for the external male to fully awaken femininity. (Note: This is also applicable to the **LBGTQ** population, respectively.) Sexual stimulation is completely "inward" and had profound capacity to open doors into deep bliss. In its essence, meditation is an inward journey that blooms while being connected to the external world (i.e. people, places, and things). As a result, the division between the inward and external begins to dissolve due to dissolution of fear, anger, and other negative emotions. The fusion of polar sex energy destroys negative energy and opens the door into pure joy. Joy is state of non-polarity. In life, most people only get glimpses of *this* joy. Once sex energy is fused, it **transmutes** into pure joy. An individual within whom polar sex energy is fused becomes a natural transmitter of undiluted compassion, unbounded forgiveness, and love without boundary. One must begin with inner research to unfold profound truths about oneself and to reach a state of pure love.

PSYCHOLOGICAL TIME

Sex energy **transmutation** can occur *only* in the present, given that life occurs *only* in the present. Therefore, the ideas and practices discussed in this book are also to be realized in the present, by examining the *nature* of one's past experiences and planning for the future. The diagram below illustrates basic truths about **psychological time**. **Psychological time** is created by thought for multiple purposes, including survival and ability to synchronize with the outside reality. In examining figure 13 shown below, one can see clearly that the past exists only in one's memory and is unchangeable. The future is the remaining time in one's life and is only a potential present. The present is the actuality of one's life and staying in the present while performing activities in the present without being trapped in the past or the future is the essence of energy fusion.

FIGURE 13: PAST – PRESENT - FUTURE

PAST	PRESENT	FUTURE
UNCHANGEABLE	THE ACTUAL REALITY OF LIFE	THE TIME REMAINING IN LIFE IS LIMITED
EXISTS ONLY IN ONE'S MEMORY	PAST & FUTURE ARE BRAIN/MIND FUNCTIONS	THE FUTURE IS ONLY A POTENTIAL PRESENT

Figure 14 shown below, illustrates four major connecting aspects of inner and external reality with **psychological time**. Memory, desire, inner chattering, and calendar time are all linked with **psychological time**. The mixture of meditation with sexual stimulation enhances cognizance and overall awareness of **psychological time**.

FIGURE 14
MEMORY, INNER CHATTERING, CALENDAR TIME, & DESIRE

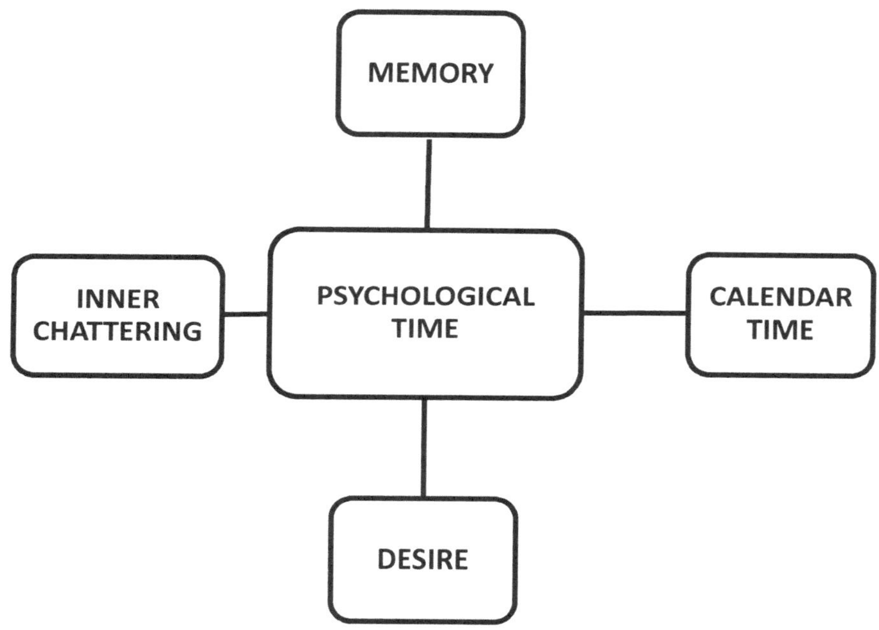

Psychological time is a creation of the human mind where the mind is generally jumping between the past and the future, without fully being in the present. Desire is a powerful force that motivates each person to perform actions in the world. Desire uses immense energy to fulfill itself and uses the intellect for finding ways to satisfy itself. The storehouse of energy *within* sexual desire can be transmuted into expansions of imagination, increased creativity, improvement of self-confidence, and enjoyment of finer pleasures. One who has strong sexual desire is seeking gratification and pleasure. Sex is one of the most powerful driving forces within the mind given that engaging in sexual stimulation causes powerful pleasure. The experience of sexual pleasure is truly compelling. It is possible to harness and mindfully redirect sexual energy into many other creative forces. One may use this energy in multiple ways that can uplift one from limited psychological functioning to extraordinary heights in life. When sex energy is conserved, one naturally begins to remain more in the present moment and not become afflicted by the torment of **psychological time**. There is the possibility of prodigious inner and outward wealth accumulating due to sex energy conservation and **transmutation**. Energy always requires an outlet and in most people, the outlet, with regards to sex, is via peak orgasms (especially in men). Yet, the outlet of sexual energy does not always have to be in a peak ejaculatory orgasm (in men) or a deep orgasm in women after having multiple orgasms. It can be given many other expressions that can open dimensions of pleasure and joy in multiple areas of one's life. Most people generally think of sex merely in a physical sense, but there are many other possibilities regarding the use of sex energy. The direction of sex energy flow affects one's: **inner-chattering**; level of involvement in **psychological time**; level of entrapment in one's own memories; and perception of calendar time.

> ***There is nothing more precious in life than time. Once it is gone, it <u>never</u> comes back. Sex energy activation throws one into the present moment. Mixing meditation with sex stimulation keeps one in the present moment. Sex energy transmutation is living an ecstatic life in total balance.***
>
> ***-- Sachin J. Karnik***

> ***Inner chattering (i.e. self-talk) diminishes when orgasmic experiences commence. Mastery of orgasmic energy reduces the frequency of inner chattering, resulting in energy conservation. This conservation strengthens the mind due to energy crystallization where the mind is merely used as a tool and not constantly switched on. Are you the mind or are you different from the mind? If you are different from your mind, then you are the master, and the mind is your tool. Intelligent and beneficial use of this tool is possible when energy crystalizes within oneself.***
>
> ***-- Sachin J. Karnik***

<u>CHAPTER 7</u>

ORGASMIC ENERGY & SEX ENERGY TRANSMUTATION VIA PRE-ORGASMIC SEXUAL PRACTICES

<u>WARNING STATEMENT</u>

This section presents material that is adult in nature.
Anyone under the age of 18 is restricted from reading this material.

This chapter illustrates a variety of sexual practices. If you are suffering from <u>any</u> physical, psychological, emotional, or other type of problem, please consult with your medical professional, psychotherapist, or other physical/mental health professional <u>before</u> attempting any practices shown in this chapter. The author is not responsible for any problems that may arise from the performance of the practices described. If you are unsure of the methods described, please schedule a consultation with the author or a sex therapist for further clarification before attempting any of these practices. Additionally, the techniques described are an attempt to mix meditation with sexual stimulation for the purpose of overall health and wellbeing. If you are uncomfortable with these practices or if you feel that the material contained herein offends you, you are advised to not read this chapter and/or any other sections of this book that you may find unacceptable. This chapter is written as an attempt to provide a doorway for personal exploration of one's own sexual energies and processes, and the author is not responsible for any physical, psychological, or relational problems that may occur due to the practice of the exercises shown

TARGET AUDIENCE

This section is specifically written for a majority of the target audience that consists of 5 groups:

1) *This chapter is for* all men who are having ejaculatory sex regularly.
    a. This includes all men who are sexually active with their partners.
    b. This also includes all those men who are using their imagination or pornography to achieve ejaculatory sexual climax on a regular basis.

2) *This chapter is for* all women who want to assist their male partners in harnessing their sexual energies. This will help women achieve multiple orgasms through prolonging love-making sessions.

3) *This chapter is for* men who are trying hard to sublimate their sexual energies (using the traditional spiritual paths shown in Chapter 4). When a man vacillates between intense sexual suppression and sexual activity that results in ejaculation, this oscillating process causes a substantial loss of sexual energy. The techniques shown here can be very helpful to these individuals who have deeply ingrained desire for sexual pleasure and are unable to adequately sublimate their sexual energy.

4) *This chapter is for* all students and practitioners of meditative sex or what is known as tantric sex. Many individuals and couples who have been practicing tantric sex can enhance their understanding of tantra and obtain a deeper understanding of the nature, structure, function, and power of the **mini-orgasmic current**. This term, "**mini-orgasmic current**" was created by the author to distinguish between the usual ejaculatory orgasm and a mini-orgasm.

5) *Finally, this chapter is also for those who are extremely serious about achieving "complete **brahmacharya** using sex."* **Brahmacharya**, here, refers to: A state of sexual function where all sexual energies are continuously transformed and not one drop of semen is discharged from the male body while experiencing multiple whole-body orgasms. A state of **brahmacharya** is also possible for women using similar practices if they avoid the "final orgasm" as discussed in Chapter 3.

> ***Meditative sexual stimulation awakens profound truths about desire, pleasure, and energy refinement that opens limitless possibilities.***
> ***-- Sachin J. Karnik***

SEX & PSYCHO-SPIRITUAL AWAKENING

Chapter 4 discussed non-sexual approaches for sex sublimation. For those who are having sex regularly and want more pleasure from their sexual activities, this chapter provides powerful approaches for unlocking one's own potent sexual power. Contemplating the possibilities for such unlocking is the first step. Within one's own sexual power exist magnificent possibilities of enhancing physical health, mental health, intellectual functioning, emotional health, and other aspects of one's life. This chapter explains how to utilize sexual stimulation for the purpose of unlocking and rejuvenating pleasure. Such unlocking and rejuvenating can ultimately result in profound psycho-spiritual awakening with many other benefits.

Historically, many traditions and societies have viewed sexual desire as an enemy of spiritual awakening or at least, a major hindrance/obstacle. Nonetheless, it is possible for sexual desire itself to remain <u>intact</u> by practicing a mixture of meditation techniques with sexual stimulation to enhance one's overall biopsychosocial and spiritual progress. This is possible when sex energy is understood and harnessed in a meaningful and emotionally satisfying way. In the author's opinion, this intelligent harnessing can be significantly responsible for excellent physical health, good emotional balance, and healthy relationships between couples. One of the major problems in married life (or any other type of intimate relationship apart from marriage) is the problem of one or both partners being sexually dissatisfied due to not experiencing a deeper erotic connection. This lack of connection is quite often characterized by, "*wham, bam, thank you ma'am.*" In the author's opinion, this dissatisfaction can be eliminated by utilizing intelligent techniques for cultivating, preserving, and transforming sexual energies and sexual essences.

EMBRACING SEXUAL PLEASURE

The pursuit of pleasure is naturally/instinctually programmed inside each person's brain/mind. The practices shown in this chapter start with the viewpoint that one can completely embrace sexual pleasure and not engage in battle with it by trying to suppress it or by trying to over-power it, as many have tried to do for thousands of years with extremely limited success. A major purpose of the practices described is to become completely aware of the nature, structure, function, dimensions, and depth of the entire sexual process within oneself. This profound awareness brings *freedom to* the sex act and *freedom from* the unwanted consequences of heavy losses of sex energy through ejaculation for men, and *freedom from* the dissatisfaction in women that occurs from not experiencing multiple orgasms.

Multiple orgasms in women are possible and can release potent pleasure naturally. Many women want to experience multiple orgasms to achieve deep sexual satisfaction. This experience of potent pleasure can occur naturally without the need for illegal drugs or other harmful substances with devastating effects. In a heterosexual relationship, female multiple orgasms become possible in the process of aiding and assisting the male partner in cultivating his sexual energies and gradually becoming multi-orgasmic. As a male partner's cultivation of sexual energy increases, the female partner can keep him interested and then enter into her own orgasms. Orgasm, as discussed in chapter 6, can be thought of as a "non-dual" psycho-spiritual connection between male and female sex energies. A man has his male sexual energy and female sexual energy. A woman has her female sexual energy and male sexual energy. Therefore, orgasm is a point of combination of (connection of, or oneness of) *both energies* within the neurobiological system, neuropsychological system, and psycho-spiritual system of each person. A genital orgasm in men, as discussed in Chapter 1, is merely an initial glimpse of this oneness between internal male and female energies. If women only have one orgasm or just a few orgasmic pleasure currents flowing through their system without having experienced deeper and repeated orgasms, then they are also experiencing only an initial glimpse of a much deeper, abiding, and fulfilling oneness.

THE PATH OF PRE-ORGASMIC SEX: POTENCIES OF PRE-ORGASMIC ENERGY CURRENTS

It is necessary to clarify that if one is already doing traditional meditation practices and is satisfied with them, and one's sex life is well regulated, there is still considerable benefit in performing the sexual practices shown in this chapter. If one is following the "**warrior's path – path of control**" as shown earlier, techniques of pre-orgasmic sex can be beneficial in the possible case of a battle going on within oneself. Nonetheless, the path of pre-orgasmic sex is intended specifically for all those who have strong sexual desires as well as those individuals who are:

a) *Interested in finding a way to increasingly enjoy orgasmic currents throughout their body, in any place and at any time.* This is a remarkable experience when this level of mastery develops within oneself.

b) *Interested in researching the unfolding of sexual energies that are hidden deep within oneself.* This unfolding has great benefits leading to inner growth and development.

c) *Curious about the actual nature of sexual energies and how they can be harnessed for the purpose of physical, mental and emotional health, and ultimately, spiritual transformation.* Harnessing of energy is like a master key that opens thousands of doors.

d) *Viewing pornographic materials and finding sexual gratification through masturbation, sex toys, etc.* If you are using porn and/or sex toys, etc. to find sexual gratification by ejaculating, then the practices shown in this chapter will be of paramount importance to you. Most individuals who view pornography would like to find a way to experience orgasmic pleasure for hours. Isn't that so? Unfortunately, most men watch pornography while masturbating and usually climax (ejaculate) in less than 15 minutes. When this peak occurs, a man feels a sense of relief and a "**negative relaxation**" occurs that is experienced as satisfaction; yet there is considerable loss of sexual energy and in most men, there is a refractory period, which can be a devastating loss of sexual desire itself. Using the practices shown in this chapter, it will be possible to experience orgasmic pleasure currents for hours together where pleasure can continue to be experienced without entering into a state of "**negative satiation.**" Negative relaxation has within it the temporary ending of pleasure by an explosive ejaculatory orgasm.

e) *Being dissatisfied with their sex partner and have been viewing pornography and/or going to adult clubs for increased sexual pleasure.*

f) *Involved in extramarital affairs due to dissatisfaction with one's spouse.*

g) *Involved in other sexual situations with prostitutes etc., and still feeling dissatisfied.*

SEXUAL UNION & THE "FIRE" IN THE BEGINNING OF SEXUAL STIMULATION

One major goal of pre-orgasmic sex is to unfold greater depths of pleasure while accessing one's inner spiritual dimension. Great beauty unfolds in this practice if the practitioner follows the steps and allows refined pleasure to expand naturally. Within this basic understanding, the "core teaching" of the practice of pre-orgasmic sex is summarized in the following teaching (**sutra**) from ancient India:

"At the start of sexual union, keep attention to the fire in the beginning....and so continuing, avoid the embers toward the end." - *Vijanabhairav Tantra (or Shiva Sutras).*

As discussed before, a typical sexual response cycle consists of the excitement phase, plateau phase, orgasmic phase, and resolution phase. If we correlate the "core teaching" with the sexual response cycle, the "core teaching" states that one should remain in the "plateau "phase by coming close to **ejaculatory inevitability** (**point-of-no-return for men**), and avoid the **point-of-no-return**. Avoiding the **point-of-no-return** is the same as "avoid the embers toward the end." The word "embers" refers to a slowly dying orgasmic fire. The purpose of this practice is to obtain a good deal of sexual gratification by being able to experience **valley orgasms** (i.e. approaching approximately 75% of pleasure experienced in **whole-body orgasm** without going to the **point-of-no-return**), where desire re-emerges with great intensity because the **point-of-no-return** has been totally avoided. This re-emergence of sexual desire is again "the fire in the beginning," and again the **point-of-no-return** is totally avoided by the act of pure attention that is given to the nature of the "fire" (i.e. **mini-orgasmic currents** that flow through the body and mind before a full-blown orgasm at the **point-of-no-return**, in men, is experienced).

This **sutra** explains the essence of the practice of transforming sexual energy with the goal of increasing sexual pleasures and enhancing spiritual awakening. In the usual sex act, either through sexual intercourse or masturbation, when a man is at a sexual peak (climax), two things happen simultaneously: orgasm and ejaculation. In reality, these two processes are different; they just occur at the same time. In relation to this, we can easily understand that there are two basic purposes of sex: 1) procreation/reproduction; and 2) pleasure. There is also a third purpose which is liberation or enlightenment. Hence, **tantra** texts describe three separately distinct and interrelated purposes of sex: a) procreation, b) pleasure, and c) liberation.[1]

Factually, it is possible to separate genital orgasm and ejaculation in men. There is also difference between a **genital orgasm** and **whole-body orgasm**. In **tantric (sacred) sex**, the purpose is *not* to ejaculate and also *not* to enter into the full genital or **whole-body orgasm**. Please note that the word "**tantra**" simply means "woven together." Hence, there is an attempt to "weave together" sexual energies lost through the usual simultaneous occurrence of ejaculation and orgasm. Techniques presented in this chapter will emphasize that ejaculation and orgasm are separate processes, and application of methods to separate them will permit orgasmic pleasure to expand and rejuvenate itself. Also, in this state, the refractory period is significantly delayed, or completely avoided, once the practice of pre-orgasmic (tantric/meditative) sex takes place at advanced levels.

THE GOAL OF PRE-ORGASMIC STIMULATION

Regardless of the type of sexual situation (i.e. with partner or solo), it is critical to understand that the goal of pre-orgasmic sex is to experience nearly endless "mini-orgasms" without entering into a full-blown genital orgasm or whole-body orgasm where there is a loss of energies and a "**negative relaxation.**"(It is important to note that at higher levels of pre-orgasmic practice, it is possible to enter into whole body orgasms without a "negative relaxation" and without the loss of mental energy that usually occurs at the **point-of no-return** in men.) This, as you can imagine, requires an intimate awareness of one's own flow of pleasure currents. So, let's get into the basic techniques, and we will start with solo stimulation.

SOLO PRE-ORGASMIC STIMULATION

A major purpose of pre-orgasmic solo stimulation is to become aware of one's internal triggering of **orgasmic energy**. There are, of course, several types of situations where individuals can use solo stimulation. Types of solo stimulation in multiple sexual scenarios are shown below:

a) Stimulation (self-pleasuring) oneself without partner and without any use of pornographic materials and/or sex toys. In this type of solo-stimulation, merely one's imagination is used along with careful stimulation of one's sexual organs.
b) Stimulation (self-pleasuring) oneself without partner and with the use of sexual images (via adult magazines, pornographic films, etc.) to bring about sexual excitation.
c) Stimulating (self-pleasuring) oneself with one's partner nearby without any touching.
d) Sexual stimulation by partner, without the use of pornographic materials.
e) Sexual stimulation by partner, with the use of pornographic materials.
f) Sexual stimulation using sex toys without pornography, without partner.
g) Sexual stimulation using sex toys without pornography, with partner.
h) Sexual stimulation using sex toys with pornography, without partner.
i) Sexual stimulation using sex toys with pornography, with partner.
j) Other sexual situations (i.e. group sex stimulation, etc.)

Please note that in each of the above listed situations, there is no intercourse with partner, yet a female partner may be using her hands to stimulate the penis and may perform fellatio (oral sexual stimulation). Given these diverse types of stimulation of sexual energy, the basic techniques of pre-orgasmic sex are the same. In general, for men, there are basic steps that should be taken to train biological and psychological sexual systems to remain in a pre-orgasmic, cultivation mode. (Please also note that the following section is written in the 1st person where the author is talking directly to the practitioner of the techniques of pre-orgasmic stimulation.)

THE STEPS OF PRE-ORGASMIC STIMULATION & ENERGY CULTIVATION

1) **Adequate privacy & time:** First, ensure that you have adequate privacy and at least 1 hour set aside to do this practice.
2) **Clean your body:** Take a nice hot bath or shower and ensure that your body has been cleaned thoroughly. You should remove all excess pubic hair, hair from armpits, and also have a clean shave. Additionally, you should brush your teeth and use an anti-septic mouthwash to kill all oral germs and destroy bad breath.

3) **Lotions, oils, music:** If you are doing this practice solo, use baby oil or other lotions and massage your hands, legs, back, chest, etc. Put on your choice of meditation music, calming classical music, or any music that relaxes you, and perform a pleasurable self-massage for at least 15 minutes.

4) **Sex meditation room:** You will need to create the adequate environment in your room for the purpose of sexual meditation. To create this environment, do the following:

    a. Ensure that you have adequate privacy and at least 1 hour free to do this solo meditation.
    b. Keep at least 2-3 100% cotton napkins with you. This can be used to wrap the penis with a cotton napkin using a rubber band or a ring.
    c. Keep a spray bottle filled with cold water within reach. This will be used to spray the penis with cold water to cool it if required.
    d. Create a sacred place in your room where you will place at least 1 candle. The flame of the candle is a symbol of the following:

        i. Pure awareness of mental processes.
        ii. Burning away of ignorance from moment to moment.
        iii. Light of **Brahmacharya** (sex energy conservation).
        iv. Constant absorption in the attractive female form with cultivation of sexual energies.

5) **Using porno materials:** Let's assume that you are using pornographic material for self-stimulation.

6) **Start meditative stimulation:** Begin stimulating your penis using your hands. You may use oils and/or personal lubricants.

7) **Absorption in the female form:** As you continue stimulating, you will notice that there is a greater absorption of your thoughts in the female form. This absorption is occurring because the male mind is churning the **subtle semen** that exists throughout the body, and the testicles are creating the physical semen that is the gross form of the **subtle semen**.

8) **Awareness of mini-currents:** As you continue to stimulate yourself, become aware of mini-orgasmic currents that are occurring within yourself. At one point, the penis will become hard and, if you continue to stimulate, you will eventually reach the **point-of-no-return**. YOU WANT TO AVOID THIS STATE. At this point, the brain

triggers the release of full orgasmic energies and ejaculation. The entire practice of pre-orgasmic sexual practice is to come closer and closer to the **point of-no-return** while simultaneously, pulling orgasmic pleasure currents away from the genitals and redistributing them throughout the body. While slowly stimulating yourself, ensure that you are taking deep breaths. If you begin breathing rapidly and start taking shallow breaths, that means that your mind is beginning to take over and is tricking you into eventually losing your semen by going to the **point-of-no-return**. Please remember that your mind has inherently built in biologically programmed mechanisms to get you to ejaculate your semen **at all costs**. Of course, this mechanism exists as a means of ensuring the survival of the human species. Yet, the mechanism has taken over human males' minds, and thus, most men want to have increased number of ejaculations with intense orgasmic pleasure. In this practice of tantra (pre-orgasmic sex), the entire point is that cultivation of sexual energies creates ongoing orgasmic experiences without the pursuit of ejaculatory orgasm. Ejaculatory orgasm may cause reduction of mental/physical energies and loss of sexual desire.

9) **Start/Stop Technique and Hold Back Technique:** As you continue to stimulate yourself, you will be getting closer and closer to the **point-of-no-return**. The start/stop technique is as follows:

   a. **Stimulate yourself slowly**: Simulate yourself and stop several strokes before the **point-of-no-return**.

   b. **Breathe**: Pay attention to your breathing and take deep breaths to calm your mind and allow the penis to lose about 20-30% of its erection. (You may need to cool down your penis using a water bottle spray, etc.)

   c. **Notice valley orgasm (mini-orgasmic current):** You will notice that when you stop the stimulation, you will eventually experience what is known as a **valley orgasm**. This is also known as the mini-orgasm or **mini-orgasmic current**, when the orgasmic current is present near your genital area or in other parts of the body. A **valley orgasm** will occur after you have become more proficient in the start/stop technique. The presence of **valley orgasms** is a big accomplishment in meditative sex. It simply requires adequate patience and a clear understanding that rushing toward the usual ejaculatory orgasm is to be substantially delayed and ultimately, avoided altogether if one is aiming toward greater inner development and crystallization of sex energy. Total avoidance of ejaculatory orgasm is extremely difficult, and it can be done *if and only if* one is aiming toward sublimating all sex energies for complete spiritual awakening. The avoidance of ejaculatory orgasms can, given enough correct practice and time, result in a profound state of **brahmacharya,** in which ever-expanding mini-orgasmic currents continue to occur, while simultaneously sexual energies are stored and cultivated in the brain. *Brahmacharya is the ideal state of celibacy; no semen is discharged, and orgasmic pleasures are available anytime in any place.*

Note: Please do not get confused by the term **valley orgasm**. The term "orgasm" in the expression "valley orgasm" is NOT the usual genital orgasm with ejaculation. It is not even the "whole-body orgasm" with ejaculation as discussed earlier. As you become proficient in the practice of pre-orgasmic sex, you may progress to the point where you will have a whole-body orgasm without the loss of energies as you could also have in the whole-body orgasm without ejaculation. This distinction must be clear if you are to make proper progress in pre-orgasmic sexual cultivation.

10) **Avoid the point-of–no-return:** Once a valley orgasm occurs, continue to slowly stimulate your penis and approach the **point-of-no-return**. Again, avoid the **point-of-no-return** and stop your stimulation. Take full deep breaths and calm yourself so that the penis drops its erection by 20%, allowing you to experience the **valley orgasm**. The **valley orgasm** may be relatively minor in the beginning. In fact, it may be just a small pre-orgasmic current that you experience somewhere in the body. Allow this pleasure current to flower naturally and die down naturally as you keep attention to your breath. Allowing this small orgasmic current to start and then naturally die down is the intrapsychic essence of this experience and the goal of pre-orgasmic simulative meditation. This current is blissful and pleasurable. The key is to not allow the mind/ego to expand this current by pushing it towards a full genital orgasm. Moving into the refractory period after a full genital orgasm is breaking the link with the female energy within you.

Please keep in mind that the mini-orgasmic pleasure current will manifest itself naturally. Allow it to move of its own accord by keeping in mind that an ejaculatory orgasm is to be avoided. Mastery over the pre-orgasmic sex current is the real goal of tantric sex and it is THE THING that will allow you to enjoy sexual pleasures repeatedly and allow spiritual transformation to occur. The pre-orgasmic current will become enhanced in time. This simply means that the pleasure current will become stronger and you will have the experience of greater pleasure as your practice intensifies. This enhancement is possible through cultivation of sex energies.

Also, to maintain adequate balance between the physical body, mind, and the flow of the pre-orgasmic sex current, it is extremely important to do adequate exercise on a regular basis. Exercising regularly will build muscle, release tensions, and balance orgasmic currents in your system. If you do not exercise regularly, sex energy will build up, and this built-up energy will most likely be discharged during sleep, or you will lose necessary attention during pre-orgasmic stimulation and move too quickly toward the end. Please keep in mind that male sexual fluids will get reabsorbed back into the body as the penis relaxes after the pre-orgasmic sex current has dissipated. This reabsorption of sexual fluids is the way that sexual energies are cultivated in the nervous system and throughout the body. In the author's opinion, the mini-orgasmic current has a great capacity to potentially heal many physical and mental health problems if it is allowed to start and die down over and over again without entering into the usual genital orgasm. When a usual genital orgasm is triggered, and control of the orgasm becomes no longer possible due to brain mechanisms taking over, there is a significant loss of energy and an overall decrease in consciousness. Of course, this will occur during your initial practices until you are proficient in being the master of the pre-orgasmic current rather than a victim of it. You will be such a victim if you allow it to expand to the **point-of-no-return**. The word "victim" is appropriate because most men are taken over by the impulse to ejaculate, thereby causing great losses of sexual energies that could potentially be utilized in many other productive and beneficial ways.

SEXUAL INTERCOURSE & PRE-ORGASMIC SEX

Once a man has become sufficiently proficient in solo pre-orgasmic sex stimulation, he can then proceed to use the same pre-orgasmic sex energy cultivation techniques with his partner during intercourse. (This is known as "sexual intercourse with sexual continence.") This practice is done best, initially, with the man on top so that he can control the amount of stimulation. Please note that the penis's entrance into the vagina of a woman is an extremely pleasurable experience for the man, and his mind will want to go toward the **point-of-no-return** (i.e. ejaculation) due to deeply ingrained programming that ensures reproduction. Hence, it is imperative to begin penetrating the vagina slowly in a very meditative way. You can try the following techniques while penetrating:

(See next page)

1) Keep the erect penis in the vagina without any movement.

2) Take deep breaths to stabilize internal desire pushing you to move further towards the "**point-of-no-return**. "Keeping your distance from the **point-of-no-return** requires remaining psychologically steady while the erect penis is in the vagina. Maintaining the penis erect in this way results in cultivation of sexual energies. Please be fully aware that your breathing must be synchronized carefully with your sexual desire and the pleasure you are experiencing. This results in greater internal steadiness due to balanced levels of sex organ stimulation.

3) As the penis remains steady in the vagina for longer periods of time, you will notice the erection beginning to drop slowly. When this happens, begin movement again to stimulate the vagina and clitoris. In this way, the female partner will have more time with the penis in her vagina leading to greater arousal and overall satisfaction.

WHAT IF THE "OUT OF CONTROL ORGASM" OCCURS?

In terms of our discussion so far, the expression "out of control orgasm" will be used to mean the following: If you are trying to remain in pre-orgasmic sex (i.e. avoiding the **point-of-no-return**), you may lose adequate awareness and tip over into "**point-of-no-return**." Undoubtedly, this will occur at times while practicing. It's important to not become psychologically frustrated due to the tipping over into the "**point-of-no-return**." This tipping over occurs due to heavy conditioning in the mind, which is functioning in a pattern and pushing you toward ejaculation. The need to ejaculate is ingrained and heavily programmed in the mind for the primary purpose of procreation. Nonetheless, please keep in mind that orgasmic currents are separate from ejaculation. Please remember that a major goal of remaining in pre-orgasmic stimulation is to separate orgasmic currents from ejaculation. If tipping over into a full orgasm with ejaculation occurs, it is an indication that the following needs to occur:

- **Slow down!** When you rush toward orgasm, your mind will trigger a full orgasm because, in that moment, you have such a compelling need that it feels like the only thing you can do. Again, this indicates that you must stay further away from the **point-of-no-return** <u>and</u> continue to gain greater clarity within your mind that going to the **point-of-no-return** is the end. You will increase the distance from that end by continuing to practice the start/stop and hold back techniques, while focusing on deep breathing. Also, continue to strengthen your desire to remain satisfied with mini-pre-orgasmic currents. That level of satisfaction is the essence of all wisdom in meditative sex and of all sexual yoga practice, and it is essential to your progress toward greater pleasure and inner awakening via sexual stimulation.

- **Continue to learn:** Each time the mind goes to the **point-of-no-return**, it creates a learning experience. Use your mind's process and abilities to find out what exactly was happening within your inner space that caused the **point-of-no-return** to emerge as the only option. This personal exploration is an important part of meditative sexuality.

- Practice orgasmic balancing: Entering the **point-of-no-return** occurs, at times, when one's mental and physical systems need orgasmic balancing due to pre-orgasmic stimulation. The experienced orgasm will rebalance sexual energies and sexual desires so that the mind experiences a "**negative relaxation**." **Negative relaxation** is the sense of fulfillment and calmness, coupled with a temporary lack of desire, that are all experienced following a full orgasm. Therefore, in one's practice of pre-orgasmic stimulation, one will, at some place in time, enter the **point-of-no-return**, followed by a **negative relaxation**. **Negative relaxation** can also serve as a significant learning experience. This "learning" brings great clarity within one's understanding of the processes that push one toward full orgasm with discharge of semen. Of course, if one chooses to enter a full orgasm, that is entirely one's decision. Remember that your goal is choosing to have a full orgasm versus being pushed into it by the unchecked processes of sexual desire.

It is also important to understand that, at times, having a regular ejaculatory orgasm or even a whole-body orgasm with partial discharge of semen can actually be beneficial to one's psycho-physiological system. This is because one's system is in the process of re-programming itself away from ejaculatory orgasm with a greater goal of having multiple non-ejaculatory whole-body orgasms. The ultimate objective can be to open up spiritual dimensions of your being via transmuted sex energy.

WHOLE BODY ORGASM (WBO) WITH PC CONTRACTION

Using the 10 steps of pre-orgasmic stimulations shown on pages 119-122, it is possible to experience what is known as a "**whole-body orgasm (WBO)**." Simply put, the **WBO** is an intense orgasmic experience where a man consciously, willfully, and with full awareness enters into the **point-of-no-return** with minimal discharge of semen or no discharge of semen. This is extremely difficult to do in the preliminary stages of your practice. It is a cultivated skill that develops over time.

Steps to Follow: If you are interested in entering into full body orgasms, you will need to use the start/stop technique for several cycles until you consciously decide to enter into the orgasm. When you consciously enter into the orgasm, you will need to contract the

PC muscle **(pubococcygeus muscle**) to block the semen from being discharged, and keep all your attention focused there until the whole-body orgasm dissipates. The ultimate goal of this practice is to enter into the whole-body orgasm without discharge of a single drop of semen. This is only possible if one has become proficient in pre-orgasmic stimulation, resulting in the reprogramming of one's system to permit a full-body orgasm. The **WBO** is your full genital orgasm with the semen blocked. The usual genital orgasm expels semen from the penis, and therefore, only a genital orgasm is experienced. The **WBO** occurs when the PC muscle has been strengthened enough so that you may contract it at the **point-of-no-return**. By contracting the PC muscle, the semen will remain blocked and the orgasmic currents will spread through your whole body giving you a **WBO**. Please remember that the PC muscle is the same muscle that you use to stop urination. The exercises used to strengthen the PC muscle are shown next.

STRENGTHENING THE PC MUSCLE: KEGEL EXERCISES

The most straightforward technique to strengthen the PC muscle is to contract the PC muscle for 5 to 20 seconds and then release it. (This is a type of Kegel exercise.) This simple exercise can be repeated 10 to 20 times in a row, three to four times per day. By practicing in this manner, one can build up the number of completed contractions and increase the amount of time held during each contraction. (For additional exercise in strengthening the PC muscle, please go to the notes and references section for Chapter 7.[1,2,3,4])

As one begins to strengthen the PC muscle and continues the start and stop technique, the ability to block discharge of semen during the usual orgasm will develop. Due to blocking of semen during orgasm, orgasm expands throughout the entire body and hence, it is known as a **WBO**. Note: It is important to remember that the whole-body orgasm (without ejaculation) is an extremely difficult achievement. The **WBO** can be achieved only after considerable practice of pre-orgasmic sex and with an increasingly heightened awareness of how orgasmic currents move throughout one's body. Even if one achieves the **WBO**, there will still be diminished psychological desire and loss of stored sexual energy in the brain and mind. From the standpoint of intense pleasure, one will have an intensely pleasurable experience when entering into a **WBO**. Yet, there is still the fact that, in most cases, there is loss of psychological desire for further orgasm, along with loss of stored sexual energy in the brain and mind. This stored sexual energy is the transformed sexual energy known as **ojas**. (Ojas has been discussed in various sections of this book.) Note: It is extremely important to read the next section carefully and entirely as it will give the proper psychological foundation for seeing the intrinsic value of remaining in pre-orgasmic cultivation mode. This psychological foundation will develop in time as the male practitioner of pre-orgasmic sex becomes increasingly convinced about the value of cultivating sex energies.

THE POWER OF THE MINI-ORGASMIC ENERGY CURRENT

The mini-pre-orgasmic current is the crux of all psycho-sexual-spiritual practices, and profound truths are embedded within it about the nature of the following: the mind; one's desire; pleasure; individualized ego; and energies flowing through the human system. Secrets of enjoying the deepest sexual pleasures unlock when there is minimal drop in energy and minimal loss of sexual desire, both of which occur after the usual genital ejaculatory orgasm. The possibility of prolonged pleasure occurs when the pre-orgasmic pleasure-energy current is allowed to move non-directionally throughout the body without the mind's pressure to concentrate it into an ejaculatory orgasm.

Mastery of this mini-pre-orgasmic current, in the opinion of the author, has at least 16 benefits as shown below:

1) There is increased awareness of "inner chattering" within one's mind. Natural stabilization of inner chattering" occurs as the mini-pre-orgasmic current moves within subtle mental layers to clear emotional blocks.

2) Natural silence occurs within the mind and steadying of mental disturbances also occurs without the need to control sexual currents through any artificial process, such as fasting, etc.

3) Intake of unhealthy food decreases and intake of overall calories decreases due to increased cultivation of energies.

4) The secret to great physical health may exist in the cultivation, transformation, and **transmutation** of sexual essences. The sex energy current uses a certain amount of energy. The remaining cultivated energies can be used for exercising, which will enhance overall health and allow one to reduce fat, increase muscle mass as well as increase overall energy levels within the body, mind, and intellect.

5) The secret to unblocking cognitive and emotional blocks exists in remaining for extended periods in pre-orgasmic sex stimulation.

6) The secret to success in marriage (or other committed relationship) exists in deeper sexual, emotional, and intellectual connection between partners. Cultivation of sex

energies keeps desire alive and allows the use of novelty to rejuvenate sexual intimacy.

7) Destruction of deep-seated anger and frustration at the root level can occur in the presence of enhanced, healthy sexual pleasure.

8) Infusion of steadiness during orgasmic chaos occurs. Usual peak orgasmic experience occurs with rapid breathing, focused desire, and reaching the **point-of-no-return**. Pre-orgasmic-mini-currents bring an infusion of steadiness created by the mind itself for the purpose of recirculating orgasmic energies and mini-orgasmic experiences repeatedly within the person.

9) Expansion of bliss-consciousness can occur due to proficiency in pre-orgasmic sexuality.

10) The secret to developing a powerful sexual and emotional bond with one's partner is within the pre-orgasmic current.

11) The secret to finding proper balance in all areas of life is also hidden in the rejuvenation of the pre-orgasmic sex energy current.

12) Awakening of the intellect to enhance and expand cognitive functions is possible by re-channeling energy within the pre-orgasmic sex energy current.

13) Many sleep disturbances and other nighttime disturbances can potentially stop if one becomes proficient in recirculating the energy existing within pre-orgasmic sex currents.

14) Sleep can become highly meditative. This is known as "**yoga nidra,**" in which sleep is highly restful due to energy conservation. The quality of dreams begins to improve, and, at an advanced stage, the quantity of dreaming may decrease substantially.

15) Existence of blissful pleasure currents can change one's attitude in life from a negative outlook to a positive, energetic outlook. Greater positive outlook leads to increased satisfaction and progress towards non-frictional action.

16) Rejuvenation of pleasurable currents is a way to reduce hyper-focus on one's drug of choice or problem gambling for addicted individuals. Also, the mindful use of this current can reduce the intensity of sex addiction. **Sex addiction** is the desire

to repeatedly experience an increased "high" by the usual genital orgasm (in men) to the point of emotional and/or physical damage. This "high" is the loss of creative **(ojas)** energies. Similar loss of **ojas** occurs in women due to hypersexuality.

Mastery of pre-orgasmic mini-currents is absolutely necessary for all 16 benefits to be experienced in one's life. Such mastery is possible through use of the start/stop technique and the hold back technique. Inward mini-orgasms will be available, on demand, by staying away from the **point-of-no-return** and thereby allowing sexual desire to remain intact. As we know now, the extinguishing of desire via peak orgasm leads to significant loss of energy. If desire can be kept meditatively active without being extinguished, and a mini-refractory period results, then mini-orgasmic energy currents can come and go and revitalize themselves. Such revitalization causes energy conservation without significant loss of orgasmic energy. Conserved energy awakens creative processes within oneself, laying the foundation for greater inward growth as well as for success in multiple areas of one's outward life. Inward and outward life become harmoniously connected via the non-fragmentation of sex energy. Given that orgasmic experience is not denied, one remains psychologically (i.e. emotionally, experientially, etc.) open to enjoyment coming from all five senses and with a heartfelt appreciation for pleasure in every case.

In such a state, inward opening of energy occurs and can take highly constructive forms. It is similar to the careful channeling of nuclear power in a nuclear power plant to provide electricity to millions of people. Personal and direct awareness of the drive embedded within desire to fulfill itself, is part of the overall understanding of desire. The destruction of desire via peak orgasmic experiences (i.e. the ejaculatory orgasm in men and a "final peak orgasm" in women), without the infusion of pre-orgasmic meditation, does not allow for the development of greater sensitivity and revitalized intensity for mindful comprehension of one's personal energy system.

A perfect approach to pre-orgasmic sexual stimulation demands perfect understanding that needs to be set in the mind before any success can occur in pre-orgasmic sex. This perfect understanding is shown next.

PERFECT UNDERSTANDING OF ENERGY CULTIVATION

(Note that the following section is written in the 1st person as if the author is directly talking to a male practitioner. This 5-pronged understanding is also applicable to women with some differences.)

The following five points are the keys to the cultivation and transformation of sexual energies, specifically for men: (See next page…)

1) Engage in energy
2) Entertain energy
3) Equip energy
4) Equalize energy
5) End in energy

These five practices are the essence of harnessing sexual energies where the mini-orgasmic current is allowed to flower and die down. In this flowering and dying down process, there is a constant revitalization of sexual energies as orgasmic pleasures flood the body and mind. This is true mindfulness as applied to sex energy stimulation. The following is an explanation of these five meditative processes:

Engage in energy: As stated before, it is important to prepare for sexual stimulation in a very meditative way. The first step is to start simulative stroking of the penis to begin the activation of sexual pleasures. You will see erection of the penis taking place, and you will notice that your thoughts are becomes increasingly focused on the female form (via porn, via your partner, or via your own imagination). You will notice that disturbances in your daily life will affect engagement of sexual energies. That's why it is extremely important to remain in a daily routine with as much smoothness as possible because conflicts, arguments, anger, and other negative emotions will disturb proper activation of sexual energies.

Entertain energy: As your penis continues to get stimulated, the **subtle semen** present throughout your body and mind will begin to accumulate in the form of gross semen in the testicles. This accumulation is normal and must occur. The goal is to continue stroking and stop before the **point-of-no-return**, as discussed earlier, and continue to experience mini-orgasmic currents. These currents will become stronger as you are able to expand the mini-orgasmic currents and continue to cultivate sex energy by avoiding the **point-of-no-return**. Remember the **Shiva Sutra**: *"At the start of sexual union, keep attention to the FIRE in the beginning, and so continuing, avoid the embers towards the end."* This teaching contains within it the great truth that the "fire in the beginning" is the fire of desire wanting to enter a state of explosive orgasm and then die down completely. The goal in "entertaining energy" is to keep attention to the "fire" and this attention will unfold within you, creating your own innate understanding about the internal movement of mini-orgasmic currents.

Equip energy: To equip energy, in the context of our discussion, is the mindful stopping of stimulation before the **point-of-no-return**. The obsession to ejaculate must be totally understood, reduced, and ultimately stopped (if one is aiming for total psycho-spiritual evolution) to completely "equip" sexual energy for use in other dimensions of your life. Of course, this can be an ultimate goal, if you so desire. Yet, for most men the practice of stopping before the **point-of-no-return**, repeatedly, should be the goal. Stopping before the **point-of-of-return** *is* conservation, transformation, and redirection of sexual energies resulting in the strengthening and energization of the entire body and mind.

Great physical and mental strength comes from the equipping process resulting in the creation of **ojas**. **Ojas** is transmuted energy, because it is *this* refined energy that is stored in the brain and mind. This storage occurs due to the *equipping process* of sublimating the usually lost semen and returning it back to the body and mind in its subtle form. The greater the semen absorption (conservation) in the body, the greater its sublimation and storage in the mind and brain in subtle form. This subtle form is **ojas**. **Ojas** is a **Sanskrit** word which literally can be translated to mean "vigor." According to various yogic paths and ancient spiritual texts of India, **ojas** is the essential energy of the body that can be equated with "fluid of life." In fact, there is a healing tradition in India known as Ayurveda and in this tradition, it is widely accepted that **ojas** is the sap of one's life energy which, when sufficient, is equated with immunity, and when deficient, results in weakness, fatigue, and ultimately disease.

Equalize energy: This is the process of taking deep breaths to move orgasmic currents away from the **point-of-no-return** and equalize their flow throughout the body. This requires the mind the be extremely aware of the flow of mini-currents. The dawning awareness of mini-currents is the first step in equalization of energies flowing throughout the system. When a mini-orgasm occurs, take full, deep breaths and this will allow the current to die down naturally. If you do not take a deep breath just after the mini-current has occurred, your mind could easily make the mini-current expand into a full orgasm with ejaculation. So, in this step of equalization of energy, the goal is simply to allow the mini-current to flower and naturally die down as you leave the psychological obsession to ejaculate complete away from your mind. Of course, there will be a deep desire to move towards ejaculation; yet with practice, this desire will make a shift where you will *want* to remain in the pre-orgasmic range. Hence, this wanting to remain in the pre-orgasmic range is a form of devotional practice. You may be wondering, "devotional practice?" Yes, the cultivation of sexual energies by equalization is a great devotional practice. You are devoted to your own internal power that is responsible for your own existence. Hence, this power can be called the power of God. In the Hindu tradition, it is known as **Shakti**. The origin point from whence this energy comes is known as **Shiva**. In additional to countless physical and emotional benefits that result from cultivation of sex energies, it is possible to naturally reprogram one's system so that the original spiritual essence will begin to show itself.

End in energy: Making a conscious decision to end pre-orgasmic stimulation without the ego ending sexual pleasure by going to the **point-of-no-return**, *is* ending in energy with transformative processes. Once you are proficient in equalizing energies, "ending in energy" is *the* master key to sex-energy sublimation **(brahmacharya)** resulting in energy usage for many other activities. These other activities can be done with great clarity and insight due to storage of sex energy within your system. There will also be the experience of ecstasy in many other usual activities such as: going for a stroll in nature; listening to music; engaging in a stimulating conversation; contemplating deeper spiritual truths; feeling a great oneness with existence; feelings of deep love and respect for all people; and, an ability to enter back into pre-mini-orgasmic pleasure currents for hours together (if so desired). The step of "end in energy" is the most critical step, requiring the greatest and deepest awareness with mastery over the movement of pre-orgasmic mini-currents throughout the body/mind system.

Respect for sex energy is the 1st step that evolves into a deep and inward realization of the sacredness and preciousness of this immense power.

-- Sachin J. Karnik

EJACULATORY INEVITABILITY & POTENT NON-EJACULATORY ORGASMS

This section intends to explain with greater depth the processes involved in achieving a state of non-ejaculatory orgasms without ejaculation. Although it is especially written for men, it will be beneficial for women to also read this section, especially if they are assisting their male partners in mastering pre-orgasmic sex. Mastery of ejaculatory control provides increasing pleasurable pre-orgasmic states and women can assist their male partner in achieving such mastery, and bring enhanced pleasure to both partners.

From what has already been presented in this book about pre-orgasmic sex, tantric sex, and the possibility of separating ejaculation from orgasm, presented here is an advanced aspect of pre-orgasmic sex where men can get extremely close to ejaculatory inevitability and stop all stimulation. While stopping all stimulation and allowing sex organ muscles to relax and again stimulating the penis to get close to ejaculatory inevitability, a man can simultaneously remain in the plateau stage for extended periods of time. The types of orgasms experienced in this situation are known as "**emissions**

orgasms." When experiencing this type of orgasm, where there is no ejaculation and one is meditatively hovering near the **point-of-no-return**, there is a "**valley orgasm**" that occurs where the intensity of orgasmic pleasure can be nearly 50%-95% of a full orgasm with ejaculation. To do this, a male practitioner must become proficient in pre-orgasmic sexual cultivation by being able to mentally remain away from the **point-of-no-return**. (Note: Of course, strengthening the PC muscle, as shown earlier, will be helpful. Nonetheless, the **point-of-no-return** is triggered by the male mind). By doing this repeatedly, it is possible to experience the resurgence of orgasmic pleasure without entering **negative relaxation**, which occurs during the refractory period of the sexual response cycle. A man's profundity and range of sexual pleasure can be tremendously enhanced. It is important to keep in mind that there is biological and psychologically conditioning to move towards an ejaculatory orgasm. Keep in mind that there is a great force within the brain that pushes a man toward an impending ejaculatory orgasm. When we consider male sexual physiology, there is a building up of various sexual fluids. The mind of the sexual meditator is able to redirect orgasmic energies away from ejaculation so that inner explosive orgasms can occur that are far more "juicy" than the full orgasm with ejaculation. This lushness of orgasmic pleasure is due to stabilization of orgasmic pressure and allowing one's nervous system to experience internal orgasms.

If you are a male practitioner of meditative sex and are interested in experiencing internal explosive orgasms without ejaculation, here are the steps:

1) As you begin to stimulate your penis, either in solo mode or with a partner, you will meditatively come close to the **point-of-no-return** while you synchronize your breathing with the movement of orgasmic pleasure inside you.

2) To do this synchronization, you will observe internally how the mini-orgasmic current moves throughout your body while your penis remains erect, and sexual fluids in your sexual system are reabsorbed. This will happen naturally if you remain away from the **point-of-no-return** and maintain clarity in your mind to avoid it, because you want to allow your system to experience greater inner orgasms. Again, this is possible once you have become more proficient in experiencing the mini-orgasmic current repeatedly as explained earlier in this chapter.

3) Once a man is close to ejaculating, all stimulation must stop to prevent going over into an ejaculatory orgasm. In this relaxation, away from the **point-of-no-return (PONR)**, one can again stimulate and build up excitement and *again* avoid the **PONR**. Relaxing away from the **PONR** allows the nervous system to generate internal mini-orgasms and eventually produce stronger and stronger internal orgasms where there is no ejaculation. In this way, there is conservation of sexual energies (i.e. **brahmacharya**) while experiencing inner orgasms that continue to rejuvenate themselves due to the avoidance of the **PONR**.

4) To avoid the **PONR**, keep in mind what happens after an ejaculatory orgasm. There is a great sense of satisfaction; yet there is also loss of sexual desire for some period of time, loss of psychic energies, reduction of mental strength, reduction of muscle energy, and a deep need to replenish that lost energy via eating a variety of foods and at times, over eating. (Hence, it can be hypothesized that heavy losses of sexual fluids can cause weight gain and possibly cause a reduction in physical and mental health.)

5) When a man relaxes away from the **PONR**, he can restart stimulating his penis and become more aware of various erogenous pleasures on and around the penis. Once internal orgasms begin to occur, the male body will develop more erogenous zones that will produce increased pleasure when rubbed, touched, kissed, etc. Remember, for the most part, a woman's body is already quite orgasmic. A male body can become increasingly orgasmic due to a gradual increase and intensification of inner orgasms.

6) Staying close to an ejaculatory orgasm, without going to the **PONR**, is extremely tricky. It requires internal determination to not tip over into a negative refractory period. Each time a man relaxes away from the **PONR** and then restarts stimulation and approaches the **PONR**, there is greater buildup of internal sexual pleasure that will create deeper valley orgasms. These deeper valley orgasms will spread throughout the body, resulting in the rejuvenation of desire after a meditative period of relaxation.

7) A man who relaxes away from the **PONR** many times and then decides to go towards an ejaculatory orgasm will experience a deep and penetratingly pleasurable orgasm that is greatly beyond quick ejaculations. When a man who has become proficient in doing these practices has experienced, even once, internally mini-explosive orgasms that rejuvenate themselves, and he then goes toward a full orgasm with ejaculation, such a man may not want to go back to the short-term ejaculatory orgasm to which he is accustomed.

Given these seven general steps in enhancing male orgasmic pleasures, a brief discussion of some of physiological processes involved in male ejaculatory orgasms will help further clarify the seven steps shown above. As excitement builds up in the male mind and body, **vasocongestion** within sexual organs eventually builds up to the plateau state and culminates into an ejaculatory orgasm. **Vasocongestion** is essential for sexual procreation in mammals, since this is the force that causes the hardening of a penis during an erection. (Note: The same force leads to the hardening of the clitoris and vaginal lubrication during sexual arousal. The decrease in **vasocongestion** in post-menopausal women may require some women to use artificial sexual lubricant to avoid pain during sexual intercourse. Please also note that the swelling of nipples in both men and women and the sex flush are also forms of **vasocongestion**.)[5]

A term known as "blue balls" also refers to **vasocongestion** and is defined as follows: "**Blue balls** is a slang term for the condition of temporary fluid congestion (**vasocongestion**) in the testicles accompanied by testicular pain, caused by prolonged and unsatisfied sexual arousal in the human male. The term is thought to have originated in the United States, first appearing in 1916. Some urologists call the condition "epididymal hypertension." The condition is not experienced by all males.[6] If a man, while practicing the seven steps shown above, experiences testicular pain due to the prolonged and unsatisfied sexual arousal, then it can be an indication that more time needs to be spent in pre-orgasmic stimulation that does not go close to the **PONR**. By spending more time this way, a proficient practitioner of pre-orgasmic stimulation will be very aware of the importance of not going too close to the **PONR**. In a typical male ejaculatory orgasm, that occurs at the **PONR**, the orgasm consists of two parts: a) an orgasm that is internal where orgasmic energy is emitted, and b) an ejaculatory response that dispels semen from the body. Internal sexual orgasm emissions and an ejaculatory response usually occur simultaneously. The practices discussed earlier intend to create the experiences of (1) deep orgasms with no semen emission (for men) and (2) no explosive orgasm (for women). By entering sexual stimulation with sexual continence, senses of each partner are stimulated intensely due to orgasmic energy being rejuvenated within. This happens when sexual excitation is occurring within deep layers in each partner and there is no semen emission. This is "erotic energy sublimation" in which the senses become sharpened. During the initial states of this practice, the 5 senses may become more energized due to enhanced sex energy interconnection. Such linking allows the 5 senses to function with greater harmony that results in the reduction of inner friction. Consider the possibility of deep sexual excitation that is not followed by semen emission. In such a state, orgasmic power is distributed away from the genitals and an "**inner orgasm**" (i.e. a **valley orgasm**) can occur. This is a state of sublimation of sex energy while experiencing mini-orgasms that eventually become stronger as one's meditative practice of sexual stimulation increases, and semen conservation occurs. There is a possibility that the sense of smell improves due to a nerve that reaches the zone of pleasure. When this nerve is activated, there can be enhanced connection between the nose and the brain. As erotic connections deepen with another person, there may be stunning smells that are naturally experienced due to enhanced inner orgasmic power. In advanced meditative sexual practices, some practitioners aim to have sexual intercourse or other sexual stimulation with total sexual continence. Sexual continence refers to the conservation of sex energy and also allowing it to recirculate when a deep meditative state is created. Simply put, the idea is to endlessly prolong the overwhelming euphoria of the pre-orgasmic state by: synchronizing breathing, flow of thoughts, flow of emotions; keeping attention in the present moment; and realizing that ejaculatory orgasm, however powerful, eliminates the desire for further sexual stimulation. (Ejaculatory orgasm results in a **negative relaxation** as discussed previously.) It is possible to eventually enter into a lofty orgasmic state with no semen emission. Such a state can potentially remove intrapsychic barriers between partners and lead to deep oneness. This oneness can expand into all areas of life when transmuted orgasmic energy begins to function in a refined form as undiluted joy. From this joy, actions are performed in the world with greater lucidity and steadiness because intelligence has been awakened by the conservation of energy. This conserved sex energy can be used for many other pursuits in life. Remember, sex energy is always raw. It can be used in highly creative ways.

> ***Refinement of sex energy opens extraordinary possibilities in one's life. This refinement occurs without the interference of conditioned and patterned intrapsychic thought barriers that exist due to reactions stored in memory. An awakened intellect easily finds countless ways of utilizing conserved sex energy without being stuck in these reactions. This is freedom in sex and freedom from limited sexual stimulation. – Sachin J. Karnik***

REFRACTORY PERIOD AFTER DEEP ORGASMS: A GLIMPSE OF THE TRANS-DESIRE STATE

If **orgasmic energy** is cultivated and one has been able to experience mini-orgasms (**valley orgasms**) for sustained periods of time, then a male practitioner of pre-orgasmic sex has the option of entering into a full orgasm with ejaculation and a female practitioner has the option of entering into a final full-blown whole-body orgasm. Both practitioners will then enter into a profound and deep refractory period due to intense satisfaction of sexual desire that has occurred within greater psychological depths. In both cases, there is no further desire, temporarily of course, for further sexual stimulation. This is a glimpse of the *trans-desire state* where exquisite satisfaction of sexual desire has occurred. Desire is the lack of satisfaction. A state of exquisite satisfaction of sexual desire is a temporary glimpse of a "trans-desire state." Trans-desire state refers to feeling a deep sense of fulfillment and a state of not wanting further orgasmic pleasure. This temporary glimpse of "no desire" is a wonderful opportunity to go beyond sexual pleasure completely, if one is interested in transcending sexual pleasures and moving into ecstasy and ultimately, pursuing a spiritual awakening that can result in unending pure love. Pure and non-diluted love transcends even the most intense orgasmic experiences. The temporary state of trans-desire may lead to a sustained state of trans-desire if a proficient practitioner performs meditation and yogic exercises, enjoys all that life offers, and performs psycho-spiritual practices to sustain a trans-desire state. This is a state of wholeness where the problems discussed in chapter 5 regarding psychological fragmentation may end permanently. This ending of fragmentation is a profound transformative and functional change within the brain/mind where all harmful, destructive, and divisive patterns of thought and emotion have subsided. Figure 15 depicts these truths, which one can discover for oneself only by direct experience through mindful investigation and clear observation of one's inner life.

> ***Without desire there cannot be any activity or motivation in life. Sex energy transmutation is the transformation of desire itself. In a trans-desire state of sexual pleasure, dimensions open up within oneself for the enjoyment of highly refined pleasures. This refinement opens the door way into pure and undiluted joy (ananda). When one gets a true glimpse of this joy, running after limited pleasure stops, without indulgence or suppression of pleasure. Pleasure is a reflection of true joy. The image in the mirror is like pleasure, the mirror is the mind, one's actual existence standing in front of the mirror is joy. Without consciousness (i.e. life) there cannot be any experience of life, including pleasure. Pleasure is the beginning, ecstasy is the middle stage, and pure joy is the final stage of true sex energy transmutation.***
> ***– Sachin J. Karnik***

FIGURE 15

TRANS-DESIRE STATE

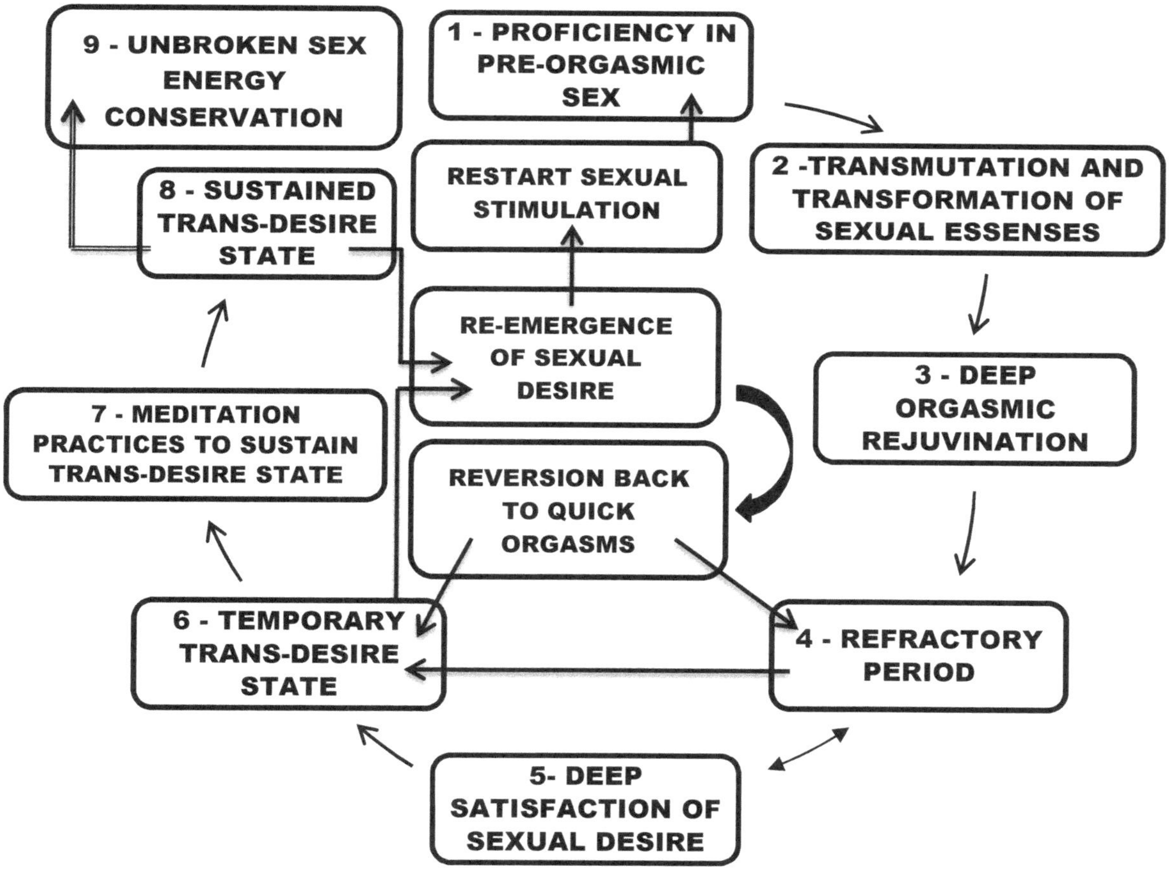

Let's examine Figure 15 carefully. Proficiency in pre-orgasmic sex is box 1. This proficiency develops in multiple ways that have already been discussed earlier. Extremely careful mixture of mindful activation of orgasmic energy and allowing this energy to be recirculated, conserved, and transmuted is a state of proficiency in pre-orgasmic sex. **Transmutation** and **transformation** of **sexual essences** (sexual energy, etc.) is box 2. Keep in mind that the word "**transmute**" refers to changing or transferring one form of energy into another, more subtle form. Sexual processes have three major essentially constructive possibilities: 1) Reproduction, 2) Revitalization of physical and mental health as well as relationship development, and 3) **Transmutation** of sex energy, which can awaken one's intellect and provide new directions of growth, where extraordinary capacity develops within oneself.

Deep orgasmic rejuvenation occupies box 3, and refers to one's ability to remain in pre-orgasmic state for extended periods of time. A refractory period will occur, even after extended pre-orgasmic stimulation, and in that refractory period, there is deep satisfaction of sexual desire. This is a period of satiety or transient sexual quiescence. This state of "sexual quiescence" is a temporary state of no desire (box 6) where there is a glimpse of a state beyond desire. Of course, this is not the actual state beyond sexual desire. It is an induced state of deep satisfaction of desire. In fact, desire is aiming to fulfill itself, and its aim is to experience powerful pleasure via peak orgasmic experiences leading to a state of deep satisfaction. If one performs meditation practices (box 7) with the aim of maintaining the temporary trans-desire state, and if these meditation practices develop into a 360-degree inner vision of one's own sexual pleasure cycle, then it is possible to enter into a "sustained trans-desire state" (box 8). Of course, sexual desire can reemerge as more time goes by and the "sustained trans-desire state" is broken when the "reemergence of sexual desire" occurs. This reemergence leads to restarting sexual stimulation and one has, again, the opportunity to become more proficient in pre-orgasmic stimulation. The jump from box 8 to 9 represents a sophisticated level of inner development. "Unbroken Sex Energy Conservation" is the state of "**Urdhva Reeta Brahmacharya**." It is a state of profound **transmutation** of sexual energy and sexual desire where orgasmic pleasure sublimates into natural ecstatic states. A state of unbroken sex energy conservation is an extraordinary state of living in which immense energy is available for personal development, growth in multiple areas of one's life, and the awakening into higher consciousness.

> ***Unbroken sex energy conservation opens up extraordinary possibilities in one's life. This is possible only when the limitations of pleasure are internalized. -- Sachin J. Karnik***

Unbroken sex energy conservation leads to inner awakening. The mind finally awakens to its full potential. Such deep conservation opens up 'divine emotion' and 'transcendental contemplation' within oneself. -- Sachin J. Karnik

MOVING BEYOND SEXUAL PLEASURE INTO UNENDING JOY

Once proficiency in pre-orgasmic sex is achieved and one is able to successfully circulate orgasmic energy throughout the body, it is possible to then revert to non-sexual meditation and prayer practices that are available in multiple spiritual traditions of the world. One may wish to do this in an attempt to move into a state of consciousness in which sexual pleasure has been transformed into ecstasy, and this ecstasy culminates, via prayer and meditation, into a state of enlightenment. This state of enlightenment is beyond all limited erotic stimulations, beyond whole-body orgasms, even beyond ecstasy. It is a state known as "**ananda,**" which is a Sanskrit word for "constant, uninterrupted, ever increasing, and unlimited state of bliss/happiness/joy. In fact, the word **ananda** is the third part of a three-part term: "**sat-chit-ananda**." The meaning is shown below:

- **Sat** = Truth, ultimate reality, the unchanging substratum upon which the world of "names and forms" exists
- **Chit** = Consciousness and pure awareness
    - "Consciousness is a non-physical entity, which is essentially different from the four basic entities of space, time, energy and matter of the conventional science. Consciousness does not have any physical attribute or property or action, but is endowed with autonomous will power of creation, retention and annihilation of the knowledge of an individual or that of the universe."[7]
- **Ananda** = Constant & unending state of bliss that is beyond even the highest pleasures.

It is important to distinguish between "pleasure" and "**ananda**." Pleasure can be understood to have a beginning, a peak experience that can last for certain period of time, and an end that provides a sense of satisfaction. **Ananda** is the state of existence that contains Original Joy, the origin of pleasure. **Ananda** is also an aspect of one's own soul (**atma**), and it is the existence of **ananda** (which is one's own self), that makes the experience of pleasure possible. The pleasure experience occurs in the physical and subtle bodies where deeply ingrained demands for pleasure come from the causal body **(karan sharara)**. The existence of the causal body was discovered by ancient mystics in India. This causal body is not really a body with a form. It is a vast collection of what are known as "**sanskaras**." These are countless impressions of past experiences that are carried with the soul as it moves from one life to another. Realization of oneself as "**sat-chit-ananda**" is only possible when one moves beyond the causal body and its countless impressions. Just to clarify, the existence of the causal body was discovered by mystics in deep meditation and cannot be proved to exist by utilizing methods in the biological and neuropsychological sciences. Via deep meditation, those mystics also found the existence of the cycle of birth and death (i.e. reincarnation). In many Western religious traditions, the notion of reincarnation is not accepted. For the purposes of realizing the **ananda** state, it is not necessary to accept the notion of reincarnation. What is necessary is to create an access point in **ananda** that already exists within oneself as one's true **Self**. The access point is naturally created when all psychological, emotional, and relational disturbances come to an end. For example, the path of tantric sex is certainly a path of pleasure, in which pleasure is not denied but accepted and naturally transcended into **ananda**. The author unequivocally believes that realizing the state of **ananda** requires all orgasmic pleasure to be transcended, transformed, and transmuted through profound inner realization of the limited nature of orgasmic pleasure-waves. These orgasmic waves cannot exist independently without the "ocean" of **ananda** (bliss consciousness). Just as waves on the ocean cannot exist without the ocean, and just as waves are nothing but the ocean, orgasmic currents are waves of pleasure on the substratum of **sat-chit-ananda**. If one wants to dip into the ocean, one must move out of the waves and jump into the ocean. One cannot enter the ocean by surfing the waves; one must move out of the waves and into the ocean. The analogy has validity up to a certain point. The purpose of this analogy is to encourage the meditative practitioner to search for the fountain of infinite joy that exists within, where orgasmic experiences are merely a pale reflection of pure bliss consciousness. To find this bliss consciousness within oneself requires engaging one's emotions and thoughts in prayer and meditation. Prayer and non-sexual meditation are a means of redirecting one's energies towards a "higher power, God, divinity, etc." Once this is done all one can do is wait for the door to open into the inner self. The door into inner consciousness cannot be opened until each and every disturbance within the mind has ended. Pre-orgasmic stimulation has the potential to end disturbances and integrate fragmented male and female energies within oneself. This integration creates the proper psychological foundation for the inner door into "**sat-chit-ananda**" to open naturally. As stated before, in the Hindu tradition, there is the notion of fusion between **Shiva** and **Shakti**. **Shiva** can be considered as "male energies" and **Shakti** can be considered as "female energies." Shiva also means auspiciousness, and when this auspiciousness is connected with raw energy (**Shakti**), then there is the possibility of moving out of limited erotic pleasures and into a state of pure joy (**ananda**).

> ***Continuous happiness is possible only when there is total balance. On the foundation of balance, pure joy can gradually increase due to inner agitations naturally stopping resulting from sex energy transmutation.***
> ***-- Sachin J. Karnik***

<u>CHAPTER 8</u>

SEX & RELATIONSHIPS

FOUR INTERCONNECTED LEVELS (ASPECTS) OF RELATIONSHIP

There are four interconnected levels or aspects of intimate relationship. They are:

- **Level 1: The Sexual Level**
  This refers to stimulative pleasure that encompasses many finer types of sexual enjoyment, as discussed earlier. The refinement of sexual pleasure can produce an adequate foundation for further growth in a relationship. The inner connection with one's partner can occur via giving significance to foreplay and to meditative sexual stimulation.

- **Level 2: The Emotional Level**
  This refers to enhanced emotional connectivity between couples leading to deeper connection. Emotion is "energy in motion." Each person experiences a wide variety of emotions and one's energy is used when emotions become activated. Increased awareness of the quality, quantity, dimensions, and depth of emotion needs to occur in an intimate relationship. The movement of energy within emotion is sex energy at work inside the emotional dimension of one's being. Emotions have a **core affect,** which refers to hedonic and directly experienced energy. Emotional experiences can be positive, negative, or mixed. This is known as **valence,** which refers to how the experience of emotion feels. Emotions get aroused under a variety of circumstances in any relationship and the level of energy or enervation of one's experience is also part of valence. Consider the following regarding core affect and psychological construction:

  > "The idea that core affect is but one component of an emotion led to a theory called "psychological construction." According to this theory, an emotional episode consists of a set of components, each of which is an ongoing process and none of which is necessary or sufficient for the emotion to be instantiated. The set of components is not fixed, either by human evolutionary history or by social norms and roles. Instead, the emotional episode is assembled at the moment of its occurrence to suit its specific circumstances. One implication is that all cases of, for example, fear are not identical but instead bear a family resemblance to one another."[1]

As stated above, an emotional episode consists of a set of components. There are a multitude of life circumstances present in an intimate relationship and it is the combination of multiple factors that creates various emotions. Emotions are "assembled" given various circumstances and energy is required to assemble these emotions. When there is good, harmonious connection between couples, the quality of overall emotions can be very positive, leading to a great deal of joy. There is uniqueness in the quality of each person's emotions given that emotion exists with subtle dimensions of one's being. The subtlety of emotion must be recognized and harnessed to reduce energy wastage and possibly stop wastage completely to attain higher levels of true intimate connections.

Emotional transformation is necessary for real harmony. Negative emotions can transform into positive emotions, and positive emotions can transform further into divine emotions. Divine emotions are beyond the polarity of all positive and negative emotions. Most human emotions are polar and dual in nature. When intimate relationship is further refined and developed carefully, emotions can enter into a divine state if psycho-spiritual practice is performed by the couple.

- **Level 3: The Intellectual Level**
  This refers to an intellectual sharing of ideas and being able to contemplate together on the mysteries of life. An intellectual connection between couples is a critical part of true intimacy. In such connection, the intelligence of each person acts without resistance and there is a wonderful exploration of life in its multifarious forms. Great curiosity about existence, nature of the universe, and many other major mysteries are explored together. An awakened intelligence is beyond the limitations of attachment with a boundary. The various actions taken by ego-driven attachment are not present in an awakened intelligence. This awakening requires energy and the capacity to perceive, without any distortion, the nature of energy disintegration and fragmentation due to conflicts and lack of non-ego driven actions. The pursuit of power is another major problem in relationships, and it creates many complications where relationships become power struggles. Such power struggles are totally antithetical to actual intimacy. Power struggles in an intimate relationship are a type of poison that has afflicted all of humanity. As a relationship becomes closer, the newness of the relationship wears off for many people, and this causes the couple to lose touch with the fresh feelings of affection that occurred at the beginning of the relationship. Ergo, there is a dividing process that occurs due to psycho-emotive saturation. This saturation causes one to feel a great deal of disconnection, leading to conflicts and power struggles. Therefore, having an intellectual relationship, in a genuine sense, is foundational for energy to flow without resistance. When energy flows in this way and nourishes one's intellect, the intellectual connection becomes solid between partners.

- **Level 4: The Spiritual Level**
  This refers to the exploration of fundamental questions about life and death, spiritual truths, and a lucid, deep recognition that life is temporary and that the time remaining in life is shrinking gradually. This recognition can lead to greater vitality. A spiritual connection between partners has three major aspects as follows:
  1) *The pleasure of sexual stimulation has been sublimated* to where the psychological drive for sexual passion does not consume the couple. Of course, sexual

pleasure can continue to exist in a relationship with an inward realization that sexual pleasure alone cannot be foundational to a lifelong bond.

2) *Great respect develops between partners* who listen attentively to each other. The capacity to listen with affection, love, care, genuineness, respect, and tolerance represents further development in the sexual, emotional, and intellectual aspects of relationship. Listening almost always involves being respectful of each other's values, beliefs, feelings, memories, and current circumstances.
3) *In a spiritual connection,* there can be joint spiritual or religious practices such as prayer, meditation, going to religious places, etc. Spiritual connection between partners is the most refined form of sexual energy. Orgasmic power has been transformed into ecstasy and ecstasy can further transform into an enlightened state.

Figure 16, shown below, depicts these four levels in the form a relationship pyramid.

FIGURE 16:
THE RELATIONSHIP PYRAMID

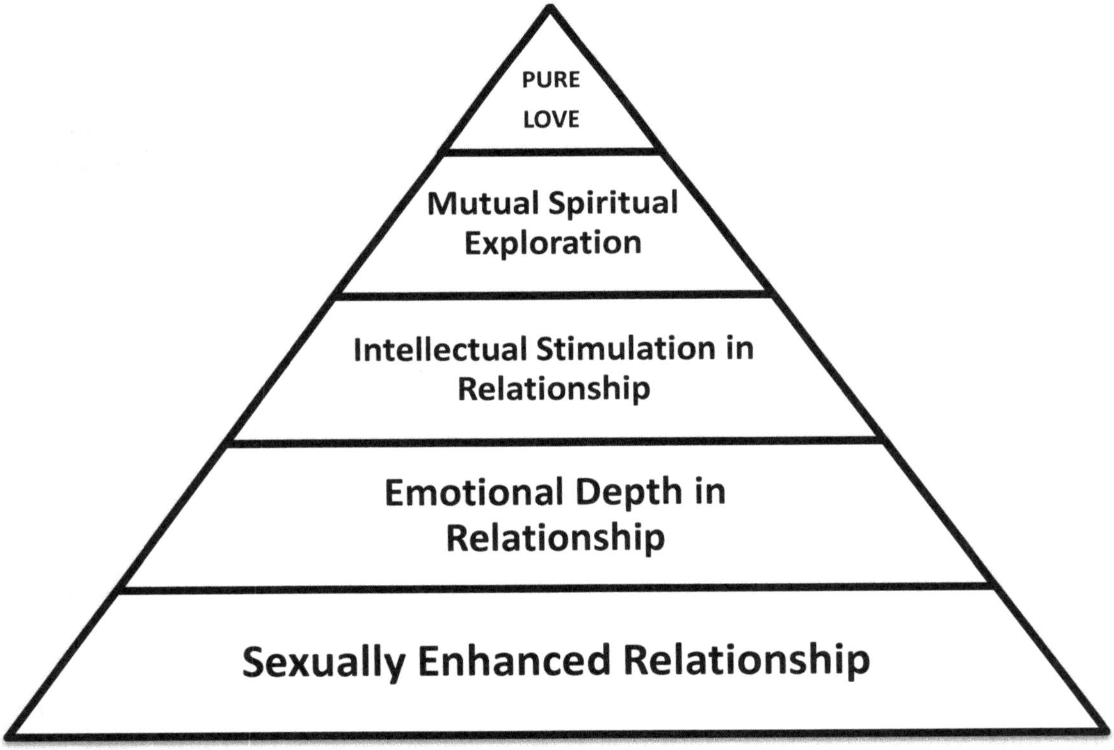

INTEGRATING ALL FOUR LEVELS IN A RELATIONSHIP

Progress in the integration of all four levels in a relationship is evidenced when each of the following occurs:

- ***Importance of acceptance of your partner without bias or negative judgment***
  Acceptance is a major component of a healthy relationship. Acceptance is the hallmark of moving out of fantasy and into loving reality. Sex has strong fantasy components to it and many are pursuing every changing fantasy. Long-standing relationships cannot be sustained when the novelty of sexual stimulation wears off. When novelty diminishes or dissipates, both partners start looking for new stimulations with other people or other forms of sexual excitation. Of course, there are exceptions to this, such as open relationships, "friends with benefits," and other open, mutually agreed upon contextual situations.

- ***Excellent verbal and non-verbal communication***
  Verbal communication is the beginning of entering into a deeper state of non-verbal communication that occurs in intimacy. Genuineness in communication is the foundation for real collaboration of two people. Sharing of thoughts, feelings, memories, desires, etc., collectively forms an integral part of genuine communication. Genuineness is not a quality that is artificially cultivated. It springs from one's heart naturally. Sex is one of the most natural processes in life, and the infusion of genuine emotion in connection with sexual stimulation enhances verbal and non-verbal communication. In this enhancement, a doorway can open into non-dual connectivity. In this state, two bodies connect, two minds connect, and two spirits connect. Actual integration in relationship is only possible with purity of communication that has honesty, transparency, and walking together as partners on the journey of life.

- ***Expression of expectations without internal disturbances***
  In any intimate relationship, there are usually many expectations. When expectations are not fulfilled, there can be considerable disturbances. The capacity to remain steady amidst unfilled expectations or partially fulfilled expectations is a strong indicator of integration in the relationship.

- ***Honesty about likes and dislikes without being trapped in a vortex of conflicts***
  Each person has a variety of likes and dislikes, and an open expression of these to one's partner without conflict is another major indicator of inward growth in a relationship.

- ***Recognition that intimate relationship is a journey taken together on the roadway of life with love, respect, and open-mindedness***
  One of the simplest definitions of intimacy is: "into me you see." Being in a relationship is to recognize that partners are in a journey together. Life is a journey, from birth to death. Existence of qualities of love, respect, open-mindedness, tolerance, affection, etc., are all emotional manifestations of deeper connectivity between couples.

- ***Relationship is the mirror in which each person can see himself/herself***
  Without relationship, one cannot see oneself. It is only amidst a variety of relationships (i.e. familial, professional, intimate) etc., that one can see oneself via psychological reactions that occur, especially when there is any form of conflict. The concept of a mirror is very interesting to consider. When you are in front of a clean mirror and there is enough light, then you can see yourself. Similarly, the quality of relationship with others, especially in intimate relationships, is proportionally related to levels of inner clarity. Staying in this state of clarity without falling back into old patterns of disturbance, is a strong indication of greater inner integration. (Note: **J. Krishnamurti** talked about relationship being a mirror.)

- ***Orgasmic pleasure is the beginning to ecstatic living***
  As proficiency expands in the capacity to master the movement of orgasmic pleasure by mixing meditation with sexual stimulation, an increase in natural ecstasy will begin to occur. Living daily life becomes ecstatic and filled with natural fulfillment without degradation of energy. The rejuvenation of ecstatic energy is an indication of greater inner integration.

- ***Deep realization that conflicts tear apart conserved sexual and emotional energies, create negativity, and reduce sexual attraction between partners***
  Conflicts destroy one's emotional and sexual energy and create negativity within the mind. This realization must occur before any progress can be made toward opening the door into real joy, which exists in a hidden form within oneself. The ability to understanding various points of view and the cognitive/emotive disposition to tolerate differences without *any* degradation of love is a strong indication of the deepest and innermost integration between partners/couples.

> ***Internal and external conflicts are reflections of each other. The source of this reflection will unravel itself via introspective meditation.***
> ***-- Sachin J. Karnik***

- ***Fantasy vs reality***
  Many men are in pursuit of attractive women, pornography, gentlemen's clubs, prostitution, etc., that can all provide a powerful experience of fulfillment of psychological sexual fantasy. When one has these experiences, unrealistic sexual expectations occur in actual relationships, and this creates many problems in actual sexual stimulation with one's partner. Pornography creates strong, unrealistic expectations regarding physical form, performance, environment, etc. The question becomes: "How can strong sexual excitation occur when one's partner is NOT as physically attractive as a movie star, model and other fantasized human beings in pornography or other venues?" To maintain newness with the same partner is possible through meditative sexual practices. This requires the "desire-connection" to remain active via "ending in energy" and not in loss of desire. Therefore, steady yet expanding mini-orgasms are required to create deep satisfaction (satiety), while keeping sexual-desire active where one is ready to reengage in sexual stimulation. Sex desire can remain active if men can mindfully avoid the **point-of-no-return** within themselves. This avoidance is done meditatively and intelligently, based on clear inner recognition and realization that activating the **point-of-no-return** is actual breakage of contact between male/female energies after an ejaculatory orgasm. An ejaculatory orgasm is a momentary non-dual connection only. Dealing with fantasy versus reality requires committed personal experience and exploration. The willingness and ability to integrate fantasy and reality in an actual relationship can be a sign of enhanced integration of intimacy. Meditative sexuality promotes the integration of fantasy and reality, leading one to real joy and not being trapped in cyclical and energy draining pleasure that occurs in fantasy. Exclusively pursuing fantasy ultimately destroys copious amounts of energy, leading to degradation of overall consciousness.

True intimacy occurs when partners are immersed in each other at all levels. This immersion is a non-dual state of living as ONE with immense respect for differences. The capacity to appreciate differences is an indicator of true unity.

-- Sachin J. Karnik

CHAPTER 9

ECSTATIC LIVING & THE INWARD JOURNEY

Living an incredible life with boundless ecstasy requires taking an inward journey. This necessitates, unequivocally, stopping the fragmentation of one's energies. From multiple perspectives, it can be stated that cohesion of energy allows for a new beginning in one's life where deep-rooted patterns of harmful conditioning have finally ended. When harmful conditioning is gone, it is possible to remain in the freshness of life's daily experiences. What is this freshness/newness? It is a state of living an ordinary life with an extraordinary vision. This book has been an exploration into the opening of this extraordinary vision. Such openness requires discovering how to live one's life with authenticity. Should one take the path of battling with one's sexual energy, or should one take the path of embracing one's sexuality to find the multitude of possibilities that exist in sexual power? Throughout this book, the author has tried to encourage you to explore this question carefully, intelligently, and experientially.

From time immemorial, humanity has been afflicted with inner battles of emotion vs. thought. Even those who are on a **Warrior's Path of Control** are aiming to end these battles and sublimate their sexual energy. Again, this is a matter of self-exploration and brutal honesty with oneself. Without such deep honesty, how is one to progress out of inner conflicts? Those who choose to take a path of mixing meditation and sexual stimulation have wonderful opportunities to embrace the diverse pleasures that life offers, starting with sexual pleasure but certainly not limited to it. Enhancement and refinement of sexual pleasure can serve as a deeper, psychosomatic foundation that leads to superior balance between the body and the mind. In addition to this balance, refinements of orgasmic pleasure allow one to deeply appreciate other pleasures in life such as music, dance, appreciation of nature, intellectual pursuits, and countless other higher pleasures. The **transmutation** process is possible when one is able to remain totally in a natural state of existence *without* energy being pulled and/or torn apart. It is only in such a state that refined pleasure will transmute further into a state of undiluted joy (**ananda**). For all this to occur, one must be introspective and learn to become a researcher of oneself. This type of inner research is experiential learning, when awareness of one's conditioning co-occurs with an appreciation that life is limited. With this realization, one is able to live in the present with greater clarity that leads to inward unfolding that in turn opens doors into limitless possibilities.

REMAINING IN THE NEWNESS OF DAILY LIFE EXPERIENCES

Transformative aspects of sexual pleasure can lead to living life with true freedom. Freedom has many aspects such as: financial freedom, emotional freedom, freedom in relationships, freedom from physical pain, freedom from tension and worry, etc. Each day is an opportunity to live with newness without carrying over problems of the past. Over analysis of past problems, conflicts, etc., contaminates the beauty of the present.

Each day is like a million-dollar diamond that is thrown away by most people in tension, worry, conflicts, and a multitude of other agitations. When one realizes the preciousness of life and the beauty of being alive while embracing natural pleasures, life becomes a symphony of pure joy. Of course, life has its multitude of difficulties and challenges. The conservation and **transmutation** of sex energy opens many possibilities for handling these difficulties/challenges. **Transformation** occurs a day at a time, and more meditatively, within the present moment. Sexual climax inherently throws one into the present moment, yet, it is only for the moment! *It is not a sustained state.* Seeking transformation is also delaying it, if there a sense of doing it later. Real transformation occurs **each moment** once the right psychological foundation is set. A transformed state will naturally occur without unnecessarily delay as one realizes the significance of not postponing it. The mind is generally caught in the web of time and not living in freedom. Even the desire to immediately transform is the destruction of patience because patience and steady awareness are required for transformation to occur. Thought must become free of past problems and the tensions about the future, allowing for transformation that occurs beyond the vortex of **psychological time**. When this vortex of **psychological time** stops, one commences each day with freshness/newness/inventiveness/creativity, etc., allowing for life to unfolds *without* psychological friction.

FINDING THE EXTRAORDINARY IN THE ORDINARY

Living and embracing an ordinary life with an extraordinary vision is a state beyond renunciation and acquiescence. True balance is obligatory for an extraordinary vision to develop. Balancing thoughts, emotions, memories, and desires is *the* doorway into understanding and perceiving oneself and the outside world with its diversity. Some on a spiritual path feel and believe that pleasure of the outside world should be abandoned in an attempt to find "God" or an extraordinary state of life. Perhaps, there is truth in such a path, and it is a matter of person experience. Nonetheless, rejection of the outside world via strict control of the sense can possibly lead to unnatural imbalances in one's life. Therefore, one must live in this world with its mixtures and diversity while developing an extraordinary vision that allows for a broader comprehension of the totality of life. This vision is filled with love, compassion, truth, personal honesty, while interacting with the outside world using transmuted energy. This transmuted sex energy awakens intelligence that promotes highly beneficial interaction with others.

Constructive utilization of energy leads to overall process, while destructive utilization of energy destroys the ability to perceive ordinary life with an extraordinary vision. -- Sachin J. Karnik

EMBRACING HEALTHY PLEASURE FOR ECSTATIC LIVING

There is a deep connection between pleasure, silence, and ecstatic living. When one goes into the mountains, silence can be experienced within the depths of oneself. When an orgasm occurs, there is a different type of silence, where other thoughts (i.e. tensions, worries, memories, feelings, etc.) are out of one's consciousness awareness, and there is *just* the experience of orgasmic pleasure. As **transmutation** of orgasmic pleasure occurs, one begins to embrace healthy pleasures due to enhanced sensitivity within the mind. This is ecstatic living where one becomes "high" on life without negative effects of the "high." One realizes that silence and peace exist between thoughts because thoughts are only waves on the substratum of consciousness. Thoughts can function to embrace health pleasure where natural silence abides. It is in this silence that sex energy rejuvenates and gets stored in a highly refined form. This refined form of sex energy (**ojas**) creates ecstatic living. Hyper-stimulation of the mind creates a stimulated silence that is mistaken for real silence. Transformation from the erotic to the ecstatic allows the mind to realize its limited nature and abandon its limitations for greater realization, *without* the denial of pleasure.

THE IMPORTANCE OF INTROSPECTION

The mind is a conditioned right form childhood. Competency in perceiving one's conditioning and to be free of the harmful aspects of conditioning develops through careful introspection. Introspection is "looking within oneself" and seeing the vastness of one's conditioning. Meditation, in its essential form, is entering into a state of natural silence and *discovering* the nature of one's inner conditioning. Mixing meditation and sexual stimulation allow for one to become increasingly aware of the nature of pleasure, nature of memory, importance of non-conflictual connection with others, and allowing oneself to experience sexual pleasure without fighting with it or running after compulsively.

Introspection awakens the dormant gift of pure observation without distortion or bias. Sex energy transmutation awakens intelligence so that energy can flow without resistance. Non-resistance of energy leads to natural stillness where introspection becomes possible. -- Sachin J. Karnik

EXPLORATORY QUESTIONS

In this closing section, the author would like pose questions for further contemplation and inward growth. Please read each question carefully and have an honest conversation with yourself to explore the depth of these questions. If this can be done with another person (i.e. one's intimate partner) or with a group of people, exploring together ideas presented in this book, then the exploration process will be even more powerful. There are 108 questions for exploration.

1) What is the connection between thought, emotion, memory, and desire?
2) When the word "pleasure" is used, what mental reaction does that create within you? When the words "sexual pleasure" are heard, what changes do you see within yourself?
3) Why is it necessary to become aware of one's own sexual response cycle?
4) Why is the mixture of meditation with sexual stimulation beneficial? What is your experience?
5) What is meant by experiential learning?
6) What is the connection between breath, energy, and sexual desire?
7) What is the difference between: sexual compulsion, sexual obsession, sex addiction, and meditative sexuality?
8) What is the difference between "change" and "transformation?"
9) Why has pornography become more and more refined with regards to its quality?
10) Is there a relationship between pleasure and fear? If so, look within and identify specific situations where you see this relationship.
11) What is the relationship between the refractory period of the sexual response cycle and tension relief? What is sexual tension?
12) There has been discussion of "**ojas**" in this book. What does this mean to you in your own life?
13) Do you believe that sex energy is God's energy? Do you believe that the source of the sex energy is in the cosmos and possibly beyond the cosmos, coming from a spiritual reality or Supreme Being?
14) What is your understanding of the "mini-orgasmic pleasure current" in men?
15) How does the sexual response cycle differ between men and women? What prevents women from having multiple orgasms?
16) Why is the male brain (mind) obsessed with ejaculatory orgasm?
17) What is required for the mind to "awaken" from its "slumber" of harmful conditioning?
18) Is awareness an activity of thought or the observation of thought?

19) Is celibacy an unnatural state? Is control of sexual impulses harmful to the mind?
20) When the word "energy" is used, what types of energy do you see within yourself?
21) What is "wholeness" in relation to orgasmic pleasure?
22) What are major causes of imbalances between intimate partners?
23) How does one transcend conceptual understanding and *awaken actual contact* with personal truths?
24) What assumptions were in your mind before reading this book, and have they changed at all?
25) Can we become aware of the totality of one's sexual process rather than being trapped in limited aspects of sex?
26) What is similar and different between:
    a. The high of "sex" vs. cocaine (or other similar drugs)
    b. The relaxation in the refractory period vs. experience of being high on opiates (i.e. heroin, etc.)
27) What is a "sexual impulse?" Can this impulse be observed internally without suppression or indulgence?
28) What is sexual desire? Is desire deeper than thought and what is the relationship between energy and desire?
29) What is the benefit of avoiding the point-of-no-return? How can a female partner assist a male partner in avoiding the point-of-no-return?
30) What is your understanding of the "sex knot" and the significance of its dissolution?
31) What if the difference between the "right-handed path" and the "left-handed path" in the "Sex-Orgasm-Celibacy Continuum?"
32) As you observe the outside world and your own inner world, can you see "cupid's five arrows" at work? What, in your opinion, is the deeper significance of these arrows?
33) Why do you feel that the "path of control" has been advocated for by many religious traditions?
34) Does sexual arousal use energy? What is the beginning point of sexual arousal? What is the difference between arousal and orgasm and how does energy flow from arousal to orgasm?
35) When the word "mind" is used, it refers to: thought, emotion, memory, and desire. Is the mind separate from the soul or is it part of the soul? Is there such a thing as the "soul" that exists separate from the physical body and mind?
36) When mixing meditation with sexual stimulation, what are the major obstacles according to your thoughts and experiences?

37) In considering the word "transmutation," what is *your own* understanding of the process of transmuting sex energy?
38) What is the difference between pleasure and undifferentiated joy? Can pleasure be sustained indefinitely? Is there a state of joy that exists beyond pleasure? If so, are you ready to take a journey towards it? What is involved in this journey?
39) In doing inner research, one must become a researcher of oneself. What major obstacles can you see in doing such research?
40) What is psychological time? Where does the past exist? Where does the future exist?
41) What is the relationship between peak orgasmic pleasure and psychological time? Does the perception of past and future stop during a peak orgasmic experience?
42) What is the difference between calendar time and psychological time? Is humanity imprisoned in the framework of limited psychological time?
43) What is the relationship between memories of sexual pleasure and internal/external triggers?
44) What is your understanding of orgasmic energy? What is the origin of this energy?
45) There has been much discussion about pre-orgasmic sex in this book. Why is this beneficial and how does energy flow occur in pre-orgasmic stimulation?
46) What is the relationship between sex and spirituality?
47) What is sexual union? Is it external, internal, or both? What is orgasmic unity?
48) What is a "whole body orgasm," and how does it differ from an ejaculatory orgasm? How does energy flow differently in both orgasms? When women have multiple orgasms, how much energy is used in these orgasms?
49) What is deep respect of one's own sexual power?"
50) How does one break out of the psychological prison of human conflict?
51) What is the relationship between sex energy fragmentation and inner conflicts?
52) What is the relationship between ego and pleasure?
53) What is the relationship between orgasm and ejaculation?
54) What is the relationship between food and sex?
55) What is the relationship between the controller and the controlled?
56) What is the relationship between the conscious mind and sex energy?
57) What is the relationship between an attractive response and memory?
58) What is the relationship between the chakra system and sex energy?
59) What is the relationship between eight-fold celibacy and sex energy?
60) What is the relationship between an ejaculatory orgasm and transmuted orgasmic energy?

61) What is the relationship between emotional energy and energy within orgasms?
62) What is the relationship between the excitement stage and energy flow?
63) Is homeostasis disturbed by frictional orgasm?
64) What is inner awaking in relation to sex energy movements?
65) What is the role of the intellect in sex energy transformation and cultivation?
66) What is the relationship between psychological homeostasis and sex energy cultivation?
67) What is psychological security in relation to sexual roles?
68) How does the identity formation process relate to sex energy growth?
69) Is sex energy movement within oneself a conditioned process?
70) What is your understanding of "sexual stimulation with continence?"
71) What is the meaning of the word "sutra" as related to sexual stimulation, and how does it have practical application?
72) What is a "valley orgasm," and how does it develop within oneself?
73) What is meant by "semen conservation?"
74) Is it possible to sleep at night without any disturbances in the mind? What is **Yog Nidra**?
75) What is the relationship between: the present moment, orgasm, and psychological time?
76) It can be said that the secret of success is to place one's mind, heart, and soul in each activity in life. How does this apply to sex energy transformation?
77) What is "unfilled sexual desire," and how can fulfillment increase without significant loss of sex energy?
78) What is the relationship between pleasure and love? Consider the following: Love is like the ocean and pleasure experiences are like countless waves on the ocean. The ocean is in the wave and the wave is in the ocean. Yet, they are still different. What is *that* difference?
79) Life is a journey from conception to death. What is the difference between the use, misuse, and abuse of energy in the journey of life?
80) What exactly is a "sexual fantasy?" How can the divide between fantasy and reality be bridge by meditative sexuality?
81) What is the relationship between self-esteem, sexual appeal, and body image?
82) What is the connection between one's physical health, sexual health, and energy conservation/transmutation?
83) Shivananda, a sage from India stated: "A mountain is composed of tiny grains of earth. The ocean is made up of tiny drops of water. Even so, life is but an endless series of little details, actions, speeches, and thoughts. And the consequences whether good or bad of even the least of them are far-reaching.[1]" How does this apply to the mixture of meditation with sexuality?

84) What does it mean to "run after excellence" in mastering sexuality energy?
85) How does sex energy function with regards to the following: "Whatever you say emotionally or with true feelings materializes, so be careful of negative words and thoughts.[2]"?
86) What is the connection between prosperity and orgasmic energy transformed into ecstatic energy?
87) How does creative power get activated in the sexual response cycle? What is the relationship between sex energy and creative energy?
88) What is your view of "novelty seeking in sexual stimulation to the point of saturation?" What is the saturation effect after seeking novelty in multiple ways? Why does this saturation effect occur?
89) What is meant by an "inward journey?" How is the mixture of meditation in sexual stimulation a mean of commencing an "inward journey?"
90) When one truly unravels the secrets of the mind, it can become one's greatest friend. Are you the mind, or are you the witness of the mind? How does meditative sexuality assist with transcending the limitations of the mind?
91) What is the connection between: the beauty of nature, beauty of the opposite sex, and pleasure? Is beauty different from pleasure or does pleasure exist due to beauty? What is the connection between the two?
92) How does conditioning occur in each human being with regards to the emergence of sexual desire?
93) Life is filled with multiple challenges. How can conserved sex energy be used to meet these challenges without the "ifs and buts?"
94) How can sex energy be used to enter the core of oneself without torment of unfulfilled desires in life?
95) What is unconditional love? Is there such a state of living? If so, how does one go from the conditional state to an unconditional state via orgasmic ecstasy?
96) Just as the lotus blossoms within the mud, how does transmuted sex energy "flower" from within?
97) Materialization of worldly desires can be possible through resetting one's emotional frequency. How can this process be facilitated using sex energy?
98) What does this mean: Sex energy transmutation is inner lovemaking using sex.
99) What is a harmful ego? What is the relationship between ego, sexual stimulation, and energy moving away from ego?
100) What does this mean: "you are the creator of your own future using the energy you have within you?"
101) What does this mean: "the outside world is a projection. Use one's sexual power to find the projector."
102) What does it mean to experience the best of life using the best energy within oneself?

103) What is the relationship between energy loss and suffering? Is there any?
104) What is the relationship between money and sex? Is money energy?
105) As it is commonly said, "nothing comes free in life. There is a price to be paid." How does this apply to the creation of peak orgasmic experiences, if at all?"
106) What is acceptance in life and how can sex energy be used to "let go" of past burdens?"
107) We are treated in many ways by different people in a multitude of contexts. Our reactions trigger inner waves of energy. How do these inner waves differ in quality, quantity, and direction?
108) *Exploration begins with total openness. Are you ready to take the journey?*

Ending of psychological limitation must occur for humanity to progress further. Although much technological progress has occurred, humans are still psychologically primitive as can be seen by constant struggle for power, position, and demanding ever increasing pleasure to the point of damaging the mind. Sex energy is the bridge between primitive human beings filled with agitations and evolved human beings, filled with immense transmuted energy.

-- Sachin J. Karnik

CONTEMPLATIVE DIAGRAMS FOR SELF-REFLECTION & DISCUSSION

CONTEMPLATIVE DIAGRAM # 1

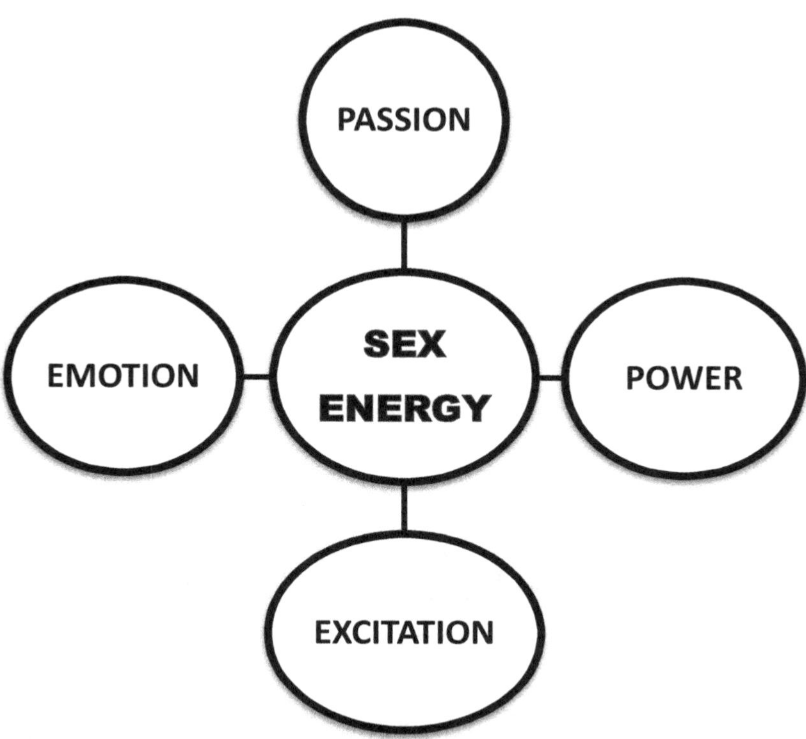

Sit quietly in one place, and ask yourself the following question and then discuss with others:

WHAT IS THE INTERCONNECTION AMONG ALL THE CIRCLES WITH REGARDS TO ONE'S SEX ENERGY?

CONTEMPLATIVE DIAGRAM # 2

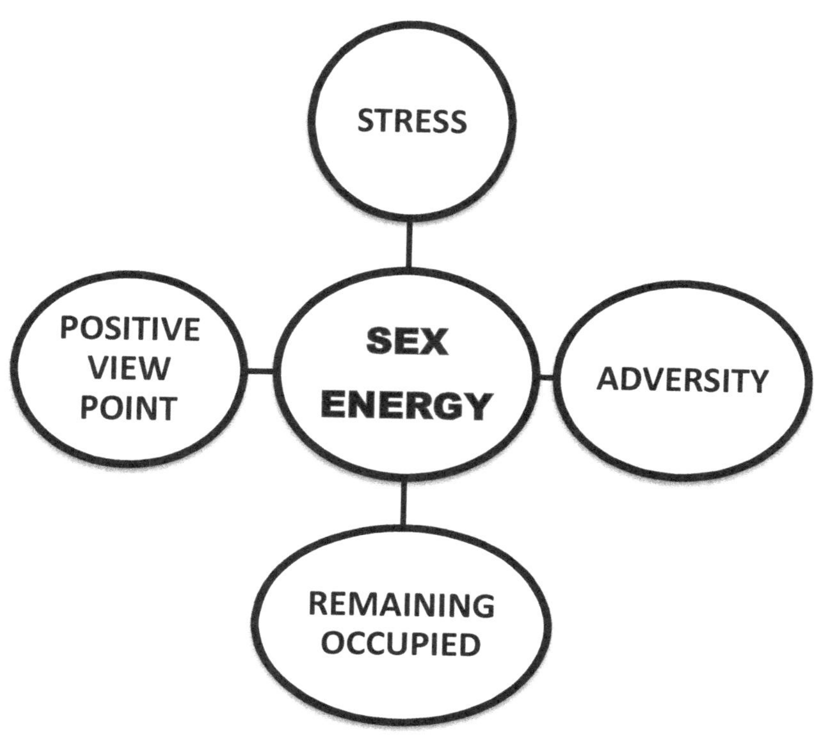

Sit quietly in one place, and ask yourself the following question and then discuss with others:

WHAT IS THE INTERCONNECTION AMONG ALL THE CIRCLES WITH REGARDS TO ONE'S SEX ENERGY?

CONTEMPLATIVE DIAGRAM # 3

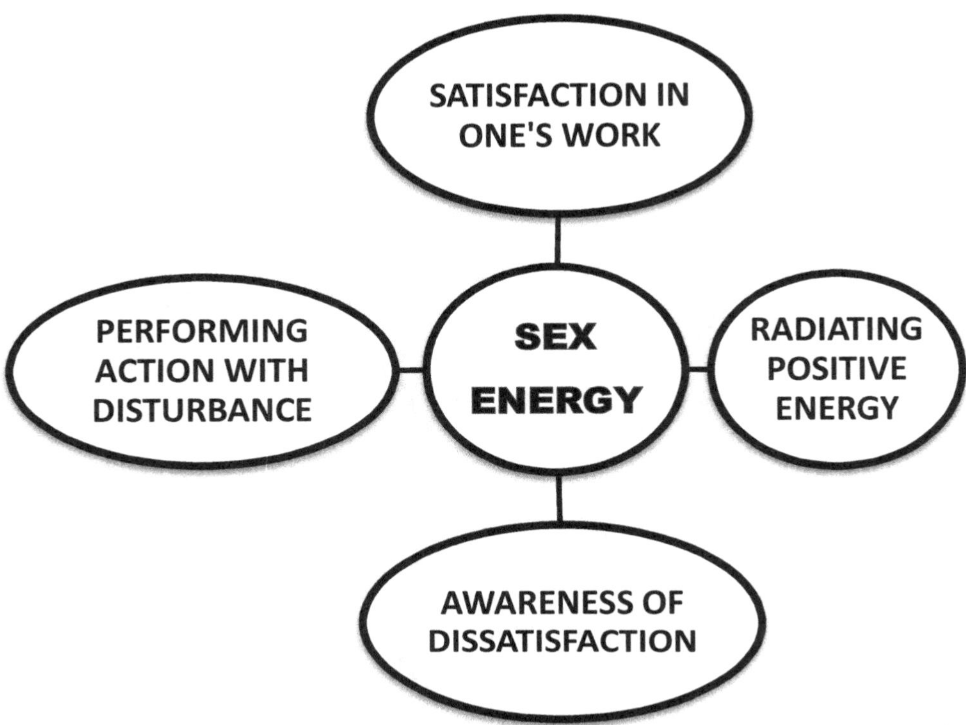

Sit quietly in one place, and ask yourself the following question and then discuss with others:

WHAT IS THE INTERCONNECTION AMONG ALL THE CIRCLES WITH REGARDS TO ONE'S SEX ENERGY?

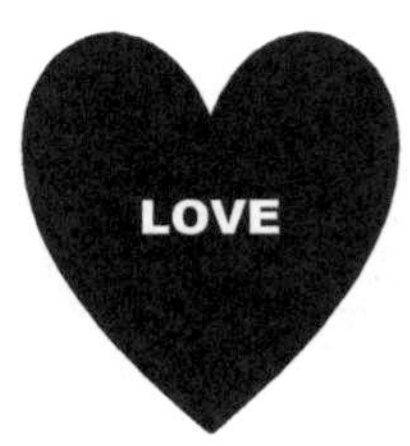

CONTEMPLATIVE DIAGRAM # 4

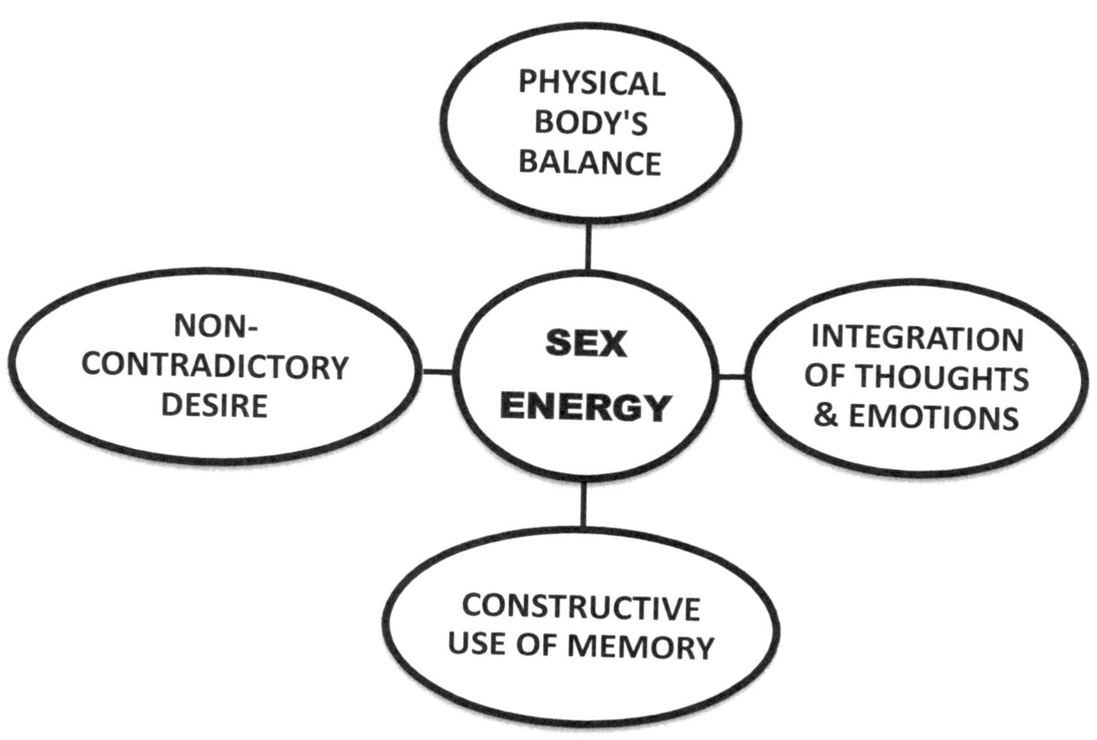

Sit quietly in one place, and ask yourself the following question and then discuss with others:

WHAT IS THE INTERCONNECTION AMONG ALL THE CIRCLES WITH REGARDS TO ONE'S SEX ENERGY?

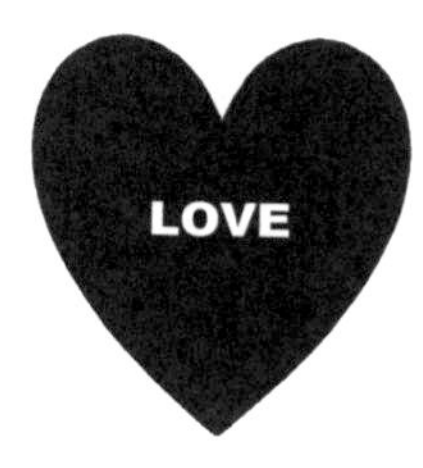

CONTEMPLATIVE DIAGRAM # 5

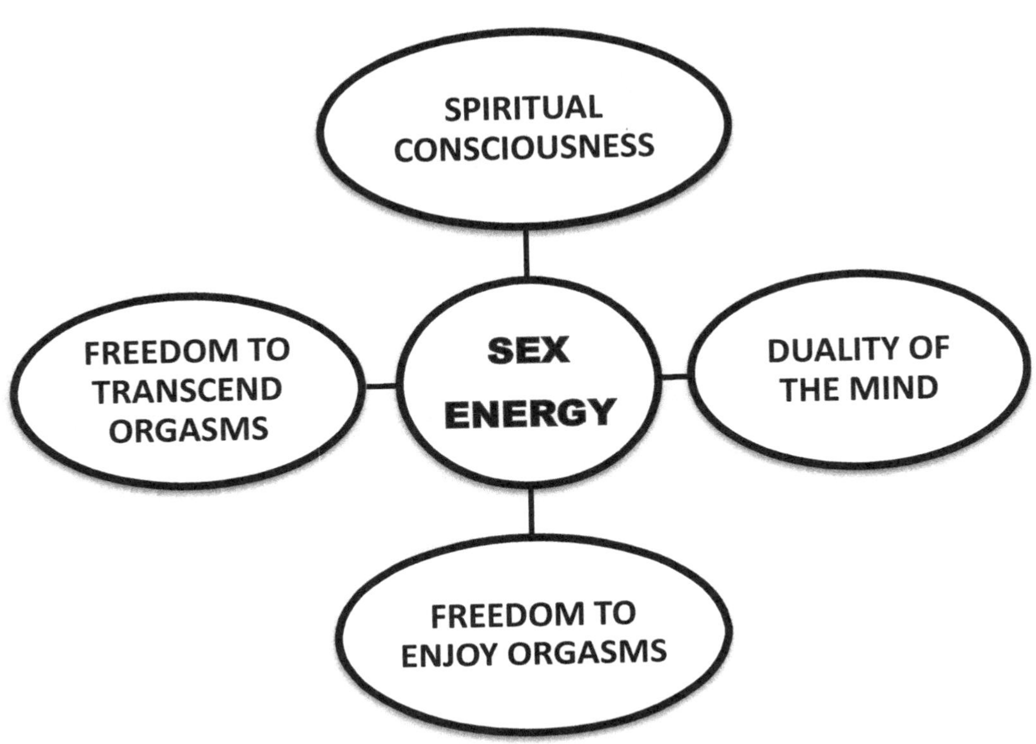

Sit quietly in one place, and ask yourself the following question and then discuss with others:

WHAT IS THE INTERCONNECTION AMONG ALL THE CIRCLES WITH REGARDS TO ONE'S SEX ENERGY?

CONTEMPLATIVE DIAGRAM # 6

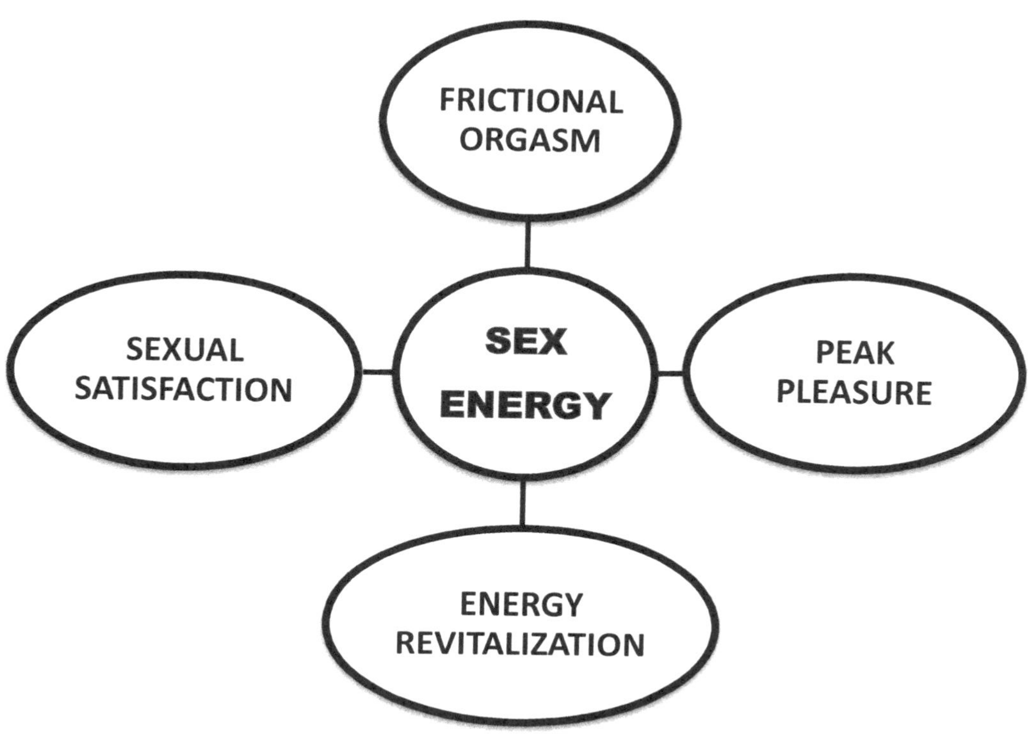

Sit quietly in one place, and ask yourself the following question and then discuss with others:

WHAT IS THE INTERCONNECTION AMONG ALL THE CIRCLES WITH REGARDS TO ONE'S SEX ENERGY?

CONTEMPLATIVE DIAGRAM # 7

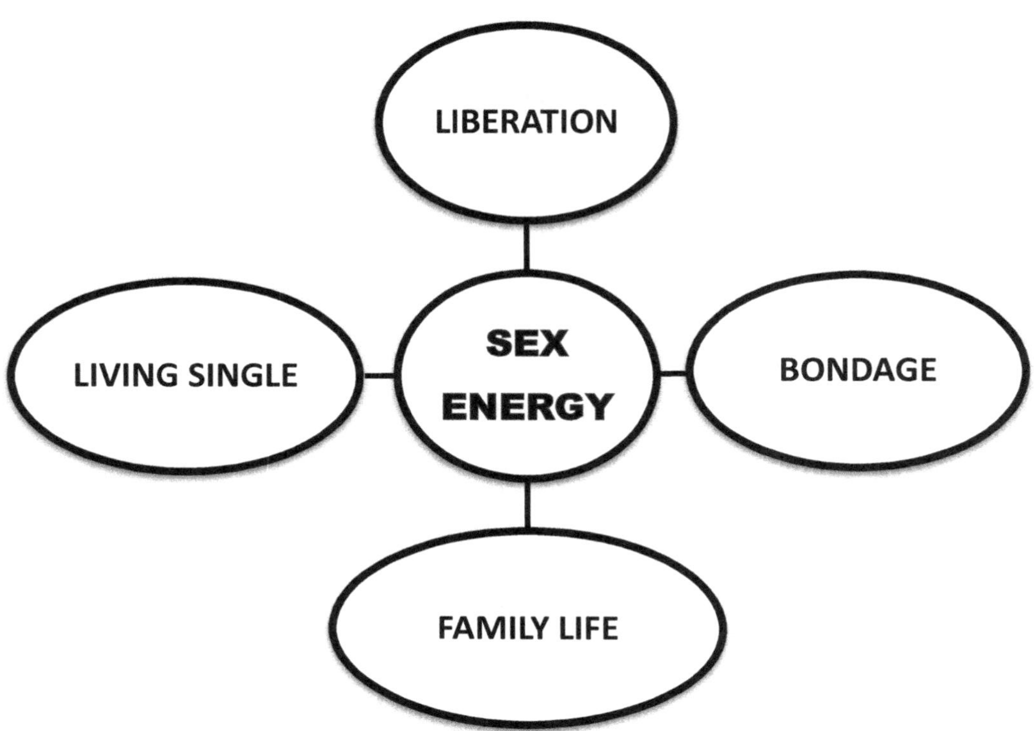

Sit quietly in one place, and ask yourself the following question and then discuss with others:

WHAT IS THE INTERCONNECTION AMONG ALL THE CIRCLES WITH REGARDS TO ONE'S SEX ENERGY?

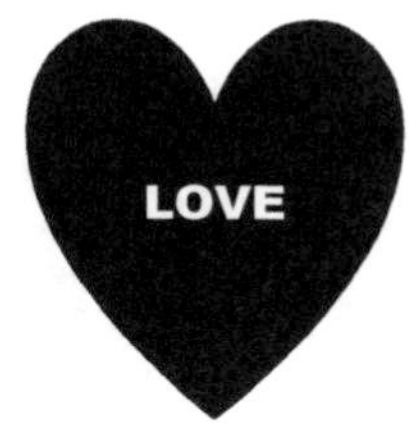

CONTEMPLATIVE DIAGRAM # 8

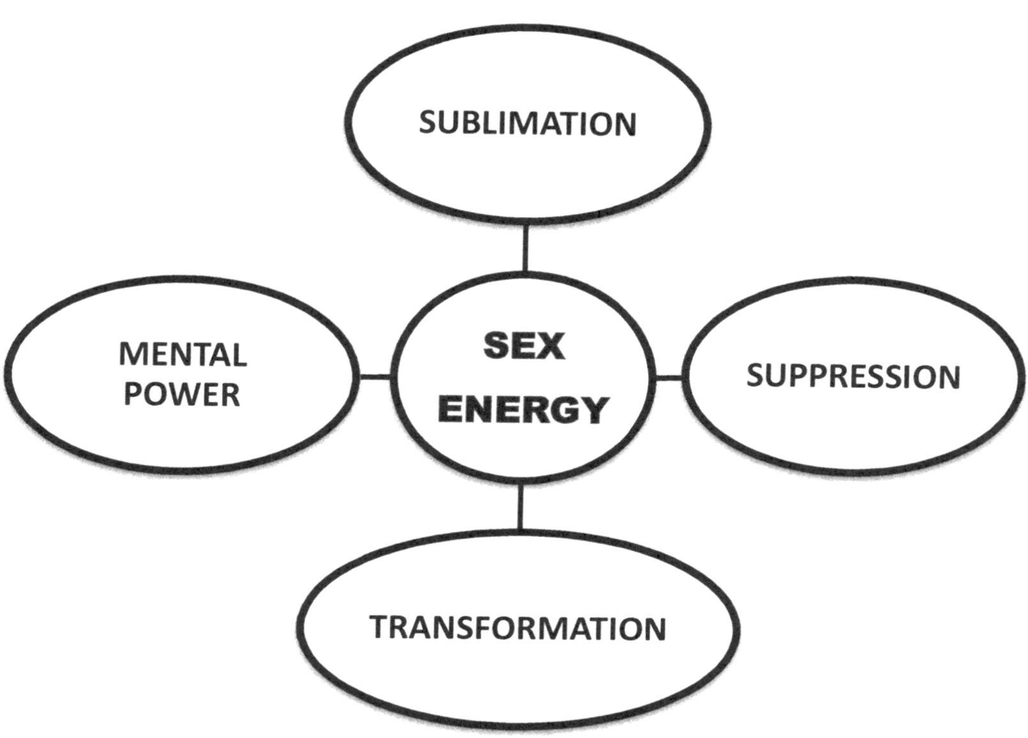

Sit quietly in one place, and ask yourself the following question and then discuss with others:

WHAT IS THE INTERCONNECTION AMONG ALL THE CIRCLES WITH REGARDS TO ONE'S SEX ENERGY?

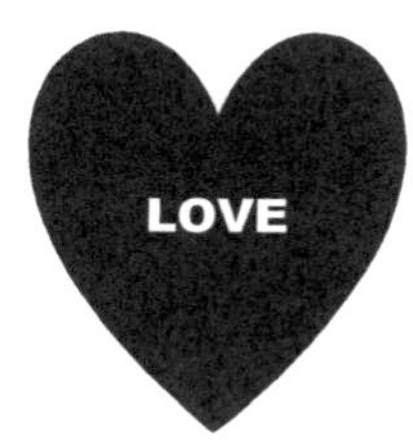

CONTEMPLATIVE DIAGRAM # 9

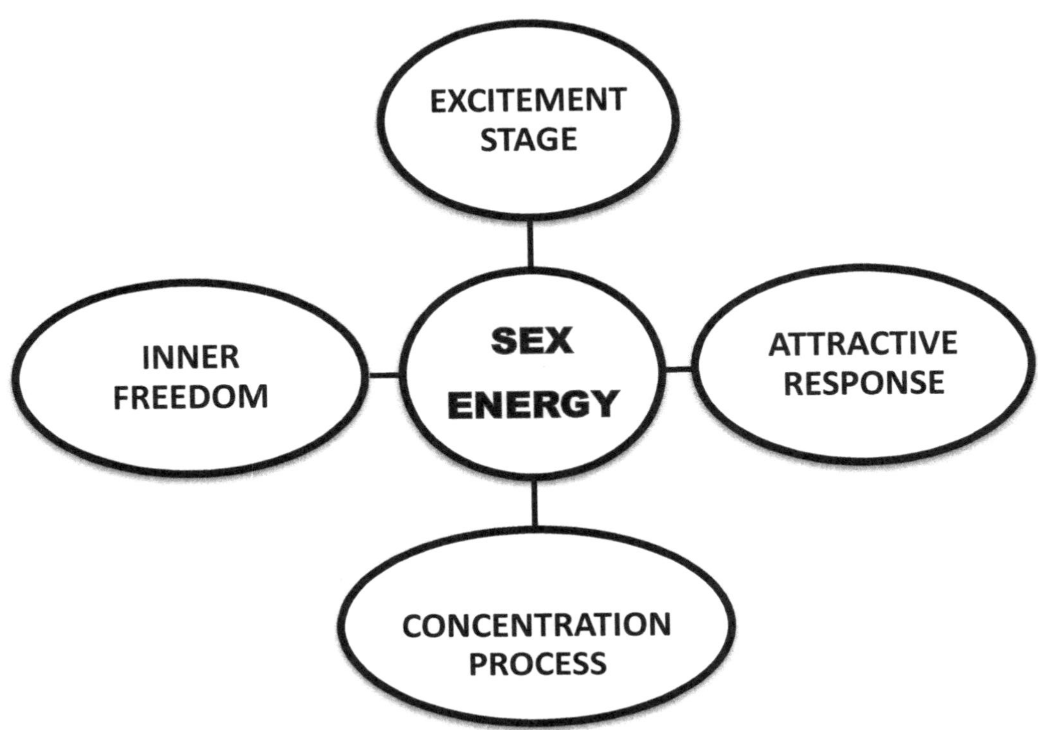

Sit quietly in one place, and ask yourself the following question and then discuss with others:

WHAT IS THE INTERCONNECTION AMONG ALL THE CIRCLES WITH REGARDS TO ONE'S SEX ENERGY?

CONTEMPLATIVE DIAGRAM # 10

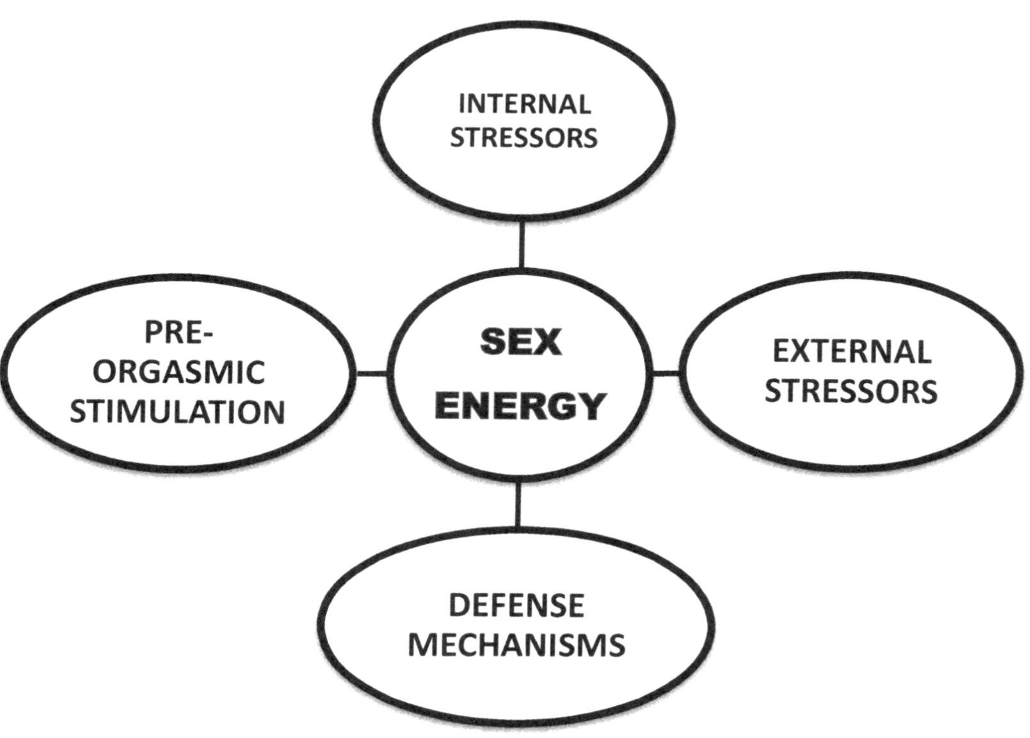

Sit quietly in one place, and ask yourself the following question and then discuss with others:

WHAT IS THE INTERCONNECTION AMONG ALL THE CIRCLES WITH REGARDS TO ONE'S SEX ENERGY?

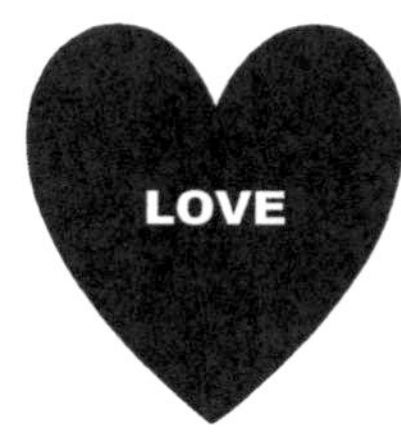

CONTEMPLATIVE DIAGRAM # 11

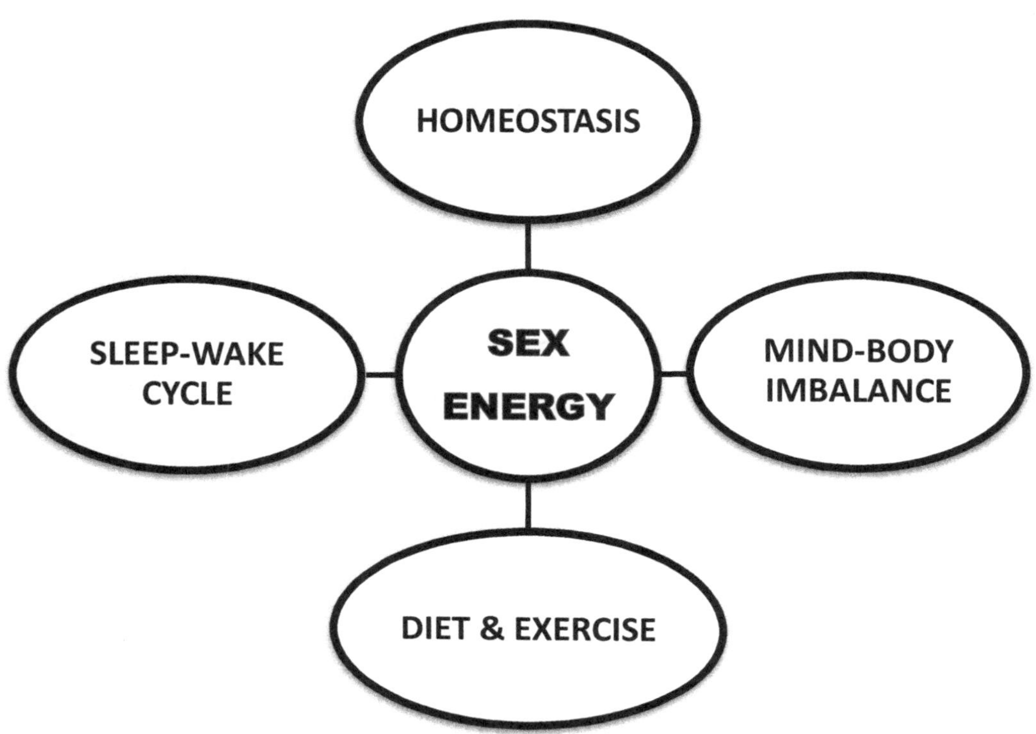

Sit quietly in one place, and ask yourself the following question and then discuss with others:

WHAT IS THE INTERCONNECTION AMONG ALL THE CIRCLES WITH REGARDS TO ONE'S SEX ENERGY?

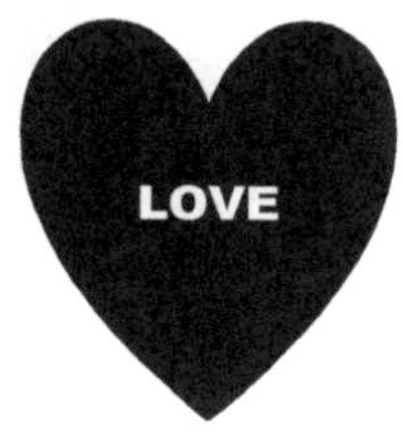

CONTEMPLATIVE DIAGRAM # 12

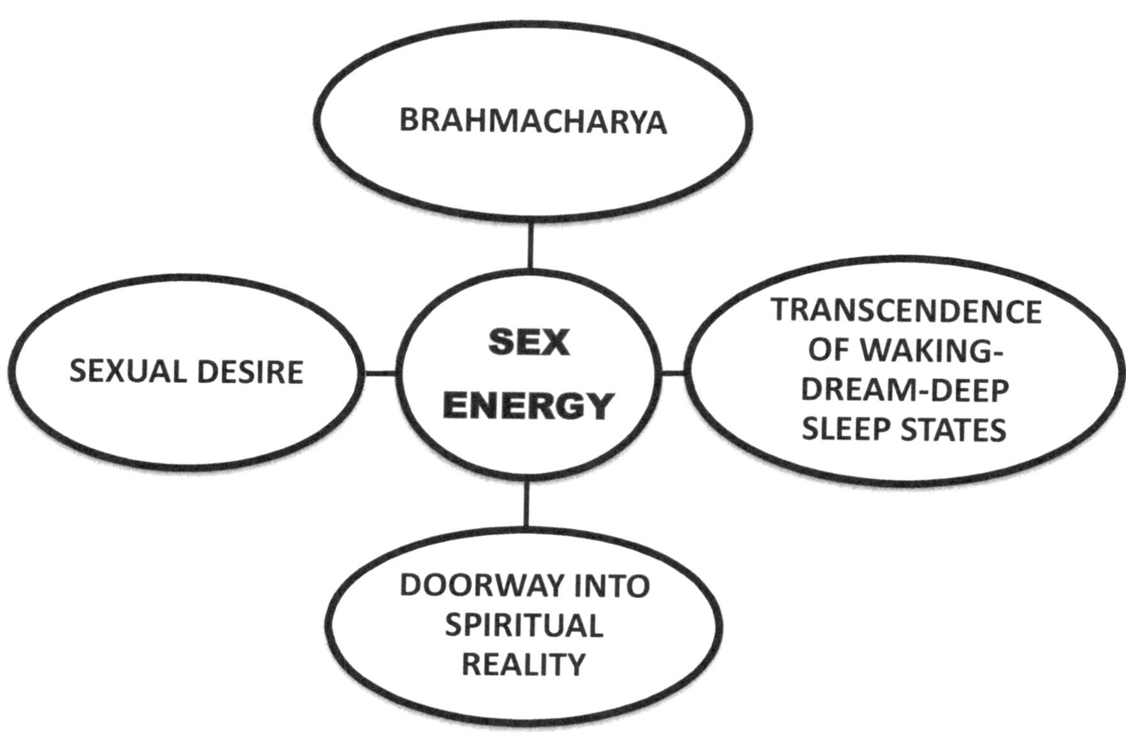

Sit quietly in one place, and ask yourself the following question and then discuss with others:

WHAT IS THE INTERCONNECTION AMONG ALL THE CIRCLES WITH REGARDS TO ONE'S SEX ENERGY?

AUTHOR'S BACKGROUND & CONSULTATION INFORMATION

Dr. Sachin Karnik is originally from India and came to the United States at the age of 8. He speaks 5 languages and has 25 years of experience as a psychotherapist. He has a Ph.D. in Social Work. He is an Licensed Clinical Social Worker (**LCSW**), Licensed Chemical Dependency Professional (**LCDP**) and Certified Advanced Drug & Alcohol Counselor **(CAADC)**, Internationally Certified Gambling Counselor – II (**ICGC-II**), Board Certified Clinical Consultant (**BACC**), and a Certified Prevention Specialist (**CPS**). Dr. Karnik is the owner and CEO of "Psychotherapeutic Meditation Center, LLC" where meditation is mixed with traditional psychotherapy to resolve mental health and addiction problems. He also has extensive study of Eastern and Western religious and spiritual traditions. Study of human sexuality has been a passion of Dr. Karnik for past 25 years from diverse perspectives.

Dr. Karnik extends his appreciation to all readers who have taken the time to read through this book. Ideas presented in this book are written at a "linguistic and conceptual" level. The real power and truth of these ideas is a matter of personal exploration. Dr. Karnik provides confidential personal consultations on the application of various paths discussed in this book. These consultations can provide great foundation for progress in one's life with regards to the conservation and transmutation of energy. Please keep in mind that this book is for the public at large and consultations are highly recommended if one is to practice the ideas written in this book.

To schedule a consultation, please contact via phone or e-mail:

Dr. Sachin Karnik
E-Mail: sachinkarnik@yahoo.com
I-Phone: 302-650-3865 (Accepts voice message and text messages)
Address: 201 Michelle Court, Newark DE 19711

GLOSSARY

ADULTERY – voluntary sexual intercourse between a married person and someone other than his or her lawful spouse. Adultery is extramarital sex that is considered objectionable on social, religious, moral, or legal grounds in many cultures and religious traditions. Though what sexual activities constitute adultery varies along with variation in social, religious, and legal consequences, the concept exists in many cultures. A single act of sexual intercourse is generally sufficient to constitute adultery, and a more long-term sexual relationship is sometimes referred to as an affair.[1]

AJNA CHAKRA - two-petal lotus between the eyebrows (also known as the "command chakra"). It is the sixth primary **chakra** in the body according to Hindu tradition. Just as a muscle can be made more powerful by exercise, the mind can be made more powerful through meditation and spiritual practices which can activate the dormant energy that exists in within this Ajna Chaka. The word "Ajna" means "command." The word "Chakra" means "vortex or spinning wheel." The Ajna Chakra is described as having "two petals" referring to a state of duality. If one's consciousness rises to the level of the "Ajna Chakra" then a spiritual aspirant is close to moving out of duality that exists within the material world. Beyond the Ajna Chakra is the **Sahasrar Chakra** (thousand petal lotus).[2]

AKSHAR - is a **Sanskrit** term referring to the imperishable, indestructible, fixed, and immutable substratum of existence. The word "Kshara" mean perishable or temporary.[3]

ALCOHOL - Many people believe that alcohol helps in coping with tricky situations, troubling emotions, and that it reduces stress or relieve anxiety, but alcohol is in fact associated with a range of mental health problems including depression, anxiety, risk-taking behavior, personality disorders and schizophrenia.
The effects of alcohol are balanced between its suppressive effects on sexual physiology, which will decrease sexual activity, and its suppression of psychological inhibitions, which may increase the desire for sex. Alcohol is a depressant. After consumption, alcohol causes the body's systems to slow down. Often, feelings of drunkenness are associated with elation and happiness, but other feelings of anger or depression can arise. Balance, judgment, and coordination are also negatively affected. One of the most significant short-term side effects of alcohol is reduced inhibition. Reduced inhibitions can lead to an increase in sexual behavior. Chemically, alcohol is any organic compound in which the hydroxyl functional group (-OH) is bound to a saturated carbon atom.[4,5]

ANANDA – A state of absolute joy that exists beyond frictional pleasure. A state of continuous and steadily increasing joy that abides in one's being as a result of deep inward transformation. Ananda is also considered be divine joy. In yoga philosophy it is said that God is "**sat-chit-ananda**" (existence, consciousness, and bliss solidified). According to **Paramhansa Yogananda**, **Ananda** is different from temporary joy that comes from sense pleasures such as eating, listening to music, and seeing beautiful things. It is also not a monotonous joy that is always the same. Ananda refers to a joy that "changes and dances itself in many ways to enthrall your mind and keep your attention occupied and interested forever."[6]

ANAHATA CHAKRA – is the fourth primary chakra (heart chakra), according to Hindu Yogic and Buddhist meditative traditions. In **Sanskrit**, ***anahata*** means "unhurt, unstruck, and unbeaten". *Anahata Nad* refers to the Vedic concept of *unstruck sound* (the sound of the celestial realm). Anahata is associated with balance, calmness, and serenity.[7]

AROUSAL - is a physiological and psychological state of being awoken or sense organs being stimulated to a point of perception.[8]

ASHTANGA BRAHMACHARYA – Same as "**eightfold celibacy**." (See definition for "eightfold celibacy). The word "**ashtanga**" means eightfold or have eight aspects. The word "**brahmacharya**" refers to connection of sexual energy with the Divine via sublimating sex energy where orgasmic experience is prevented. This practice is part of the "right-handed" path of sex-sublimation.

ATAVISTIC REWARDS – relating to or characterized by reversion to something ancient or ancestral. Sexual gratification can be considered as an "atavistic reward" due to the ancestral and ancient nature of sexual impulses. Transformation into higher consciousness requires reducing psychological fixation on atavistic rewards without problems of suppression and repression.[9]

ATMA - is a **Sanskrit** word that means inner-self or soul. This is the "witnessing consciousness" that observes processes of thought, emotion, memory, and desire. Many Eastern spiritual texts describe the atma as: a divine spark, the essential nature of oneself; composite of truth-consciousness-and bliss; divine light that is perceived in deep meditation.[10]

ATTRACTION RESPONSE – A response in the mind where another person is perceived as "attractive." This response starts generating some pleasure within oneself with the aim of reaching deeper levels of excitation and pleasure. Biologically, this response is programmed within the brain for the purpose of reproduction that has potent energy responsible for ensuring survival of the human species.

BINDU – is a **Sanskrit** word meaning "point" or "dot." Semen is considered to be "bindu" given that ejaculatory orgasm in the male body is a climactic point. Semen itself is considered to be "bindu" which also refers to drops. Hence, drops of semen are considered to be "bindu."[11]

BLOOD – is a body fluid in humans and other animals that delivers necessary substances such as nutrients and oxygen to the cells and transports metabolic waste products away from those same cells.[12]

BLUE BALLS – is a slang term for the condition of temporary fluid congestion (**vasocongestion**) in the testicles accompanied by testicular pain, caused by prolonged sexual arousal in the male without ejaculation. The practices of meditative stimulation emphasis brief periods of arousal and do not promote prolonged sexual arousal.[13]

BONE MARROW - is the flexible tissue in the interior of bones. In humans, red blood cells are produced by cores of bone marrow in the heads of long bones in a process known as hematopoiesis.[14]

BRAHMACHARI - a student of the Vedas, especially one committed to **brahmacharya.**[15]

BRAHMACHARYA - literally means "going after Brahman (Supreme Reality, Self or God)". In Indian religions, it is also a concept with various context-driven meanings. Brahmacharya is sex energy sublimation and transmutation where this energy flows upwards for spiritual awakening. The state of continual and unbroken upward flow of sex energy is known as "**urdhva-reeta brahmacharya.**"[16]

BRAHMANDA – The universe is called "brahmanda" in the Sanskrit language. The universe is considered to be evolved out of Brahman (i.e. God) where the "anda" means egg. Hence, each universe is like an "egg" hatched from the spiritual dimension.

BRAHMA-TEJA – This refers to transformed sex energy that has been sublimated within oneself which gives a brightness to one's face. This "brightness" can be seen on the faces of those who have sublimated the sex energy for many years. Intellectual strength and memory capacity increases substantially due to sex energy sublimation.

CHAKRA – is any spiritual vortex connected to the subtle body. Chakras are believed to be psychic-energy centers in the esoteric traditions of Indian religions. The word "chakra" refers to "spinning vortex" that has spiritual energy within it. This energy is responsible for the creation of experiences within the waking and dream state. The light within each chakra is the light of the soul coming from God.[17]

CHITTA – This refers to the subconscious mind that is a storehouse of memories.

CHYLE – is a milky bodily fluid consisting of lymph and emulsified fats, or free fatty acids.[18]

COITUS - physical union of male and female genitalia accompanied by rhythmic movements. Is principally the insertion and thrusting of the penis, usually when erect, into the vagina for sexual pleasure, reproduction, or both.[19]

COITUS RESERVATUS – See **Sexual Continence**. There is a slight difference between **karezza** and coitus reservatus. In coitus reservatus, unlike **karezza**, a woman can enjoy a prolonged orgasm while a man exercises self-control; similarly, in the context of two male sexual partners, the receptive partner can enjoy the stimulation of his prostate for a longer period of time than he would otherwise. Coitus reservatus is also known as sexual continence where a form of sexual intercourse occurs in which the penetrative partner does not attempt to ejaculate within the receptive partner, but instead attempts to remain in the plateau phase of intercourse for as long as possible avoiding seminal emissions.[20]

CONSCIOUS MIND – The state or condition of being conscious. A sense of one's personal or collective identity; including the attitudes, beliefs, and sensitivities held by or considered characteristic of an individual or group.[21]

CONTROLLED – Philosopher **J. Krishnamurti** has talk about this division between the controller and controlled. The "controlled" refers to aspects of thought and emotion that are being controlled by another thought or a combination of thoughts that constitute the "controller."

CONTROLLER – The controller is a set of thoughts that combine together to control another set of thoughts. In a broader sense, the controller is an interconnected set of thoughts, emotions, memories, and desires that function as one process to control a variety of processes within the mind.

DESIRE – refers to wanting of sexual stimulation and/or sexual contact, in context of current book. In general, desire is the lack of the state of satisfaction. For example, once an ejaculatory orgasm occurs, there is temporary state of "no desire" or "minimal desire" during the refractory period of the sexual response cycle.

DHATU – Sanskrit term for the seven fundamental elements within the body. These can be thought of as: layer, stratum, constituent part, ingredient, element, primitive matter. In Ayurveda, the seven fundamental principles (elements) that support the basic structure (and functioning) of the body are considered to be Dhatus. The dhatus are the basic varieties of tissues which compose the human body. The word "dhatu" comes from a **Sanskrit** word which means "that which enters into the formation of the body"; the root Daa (dha) means "support, that which bears."[22,23,24]
The primary Dhatus are seven in number. They are:

- Sukra dhatu (reproductive tissues)
- Majja dhatu (bone marrow and nervous tissues)
- Asthi dhatu (bone)
- Meda dhatu (fatty tissues)
- Mamsa dhatu (muscle tissues)
- Rakta dhatu (formed blood cells)
- Rasa dhatu (plasma)

DRIVE – Refers to instinctual processes that are responsible for creating the experience of desire. Sexual desire exists as part of overall instinctual drives.

EIGHTFOLD CELIBACY – This is the same as "**ashtanga brahmacharya**." There are monks (**sadhus**) in some religious organizations that follow this path of sex energy sublimation. They follow this path by avoiding contact with the opposite sex in eight ways: a) avoid touching the opposite sex; b) avoid seeing the opposite sex in a way that create an attractive response; c) avoid hearing the voice of the opposite sex (an extreme level of this practice); d) avoiding smelling perfumes or other such items that can cause activation of sexual desire; e) avoid eating foods that can activate or intensify sexual desire; f) avoid remembering past sexual pleasures or sexual acts and avoid remembering a form of the opposite sex that may have been seen as attractive in the mind; g) avoid making a determination to engage in sexual stimulation in any form; h) avoid engage in actual sexual act.

EJACULATE – to eject (semen), to eject suddenly and swiftly; discharge. This also refers to the total amount of semen fluid.[25]

EJACULATION – an abrupt, exclamatory utterance, the act or process of ejaculating, especially the discharge of semen by the male reproductive organs. Male orgasm is usually accompanied with ejaculation. Through meditation practices, it is possible to separate orgasm and ejaculation where internal orgasms can occur without ejaculation.[26]

EJACULATORY INEVITABILITY - The point during sexual intercourse where the male realizes he is about to ejaculate (i.e. cum) no matter what he does to stop it. Usually at this point semen has already entered the base of the shaft of the penis, so the male cannot stop the ejaculation process no matter how hard he tries.[27]

EJACULATORY ORGASM - A male orgasm with ejaculation. This is what most men are pursuing as a climatic point in their sexual activity.

EMISSIONS ORGASMS – This refers to "inner orgasms" without ejaculation. There can be some pre-ejaculate fluid that is discharge during these orgasms.

EMOTIONAL ENERGY – refers to the energy that flows within the entire emotional system.

EXCITEMENT STAGE – during this state of the sexual response cycle, the body prepares for sexual activity by tensing muscles and increasing heart rate. In the male, blood flows into the penis, causing it to become erect; in the female, the vaginal walls become moist, the inner part of the vagina becomes wider, and the clitoris enlarges.[28]

EXPERIENCER – Refers to the "soul or atma" that is experiencing the outside world and the inner world. This is also known as the seer behind the senses. Empiricists believe that the brain generates the "experiencer" while spiritualists believe that the "experiencer" exists beyond the mind and is the witnessing consciousness. In certain religious/spiritual traditions, there is a belief that God exists within the "experiencer" as giver of the fruits of one's actions.

FEMALE EJACULATION – is the expulsion of fluid from or near the vagina during or before an orgasm. It is also known colloquially as squirting or gushing.[29]

GENITAL ORGASM – This a male orgasm that is felt deeply in the genital area.

GENOME - is the genetic material of an organism. In each human being, there exist 46 chromosomes.[30]

GOD – Considered by many religious traditions as a "supreme being" or "ultimate reality." There are many concepts of God. Sexual energy is considered to be God's creative energy placed in each human being for the propagation of the species, according to some traditions.

HEAVEN – is a common religious, cosmological, or transcendent place where beings such as gods, angles, saints, or venerated ancestors are said to originate, be enthroned, or live. A possible psychological and trans-psychological state of being where there is total joy and possibly direct contact and entering into a spiritual world.[31]

HEDONIC SET POINT – This is the point where substantial amount of sexual pleasure is experienced.

HOMEOSTASIS – is the property of a system within the body of an organism in which a variable, such as the concentration of a substance in solution, is actively regulated to remain very nearly constant. With regards to sexual functioning, keeping sexual desire balanced is a type of **psychological homeostasis**.[32]

HOMEOSTATIC IMBALANCES – is the disability of the internal environment to remain in equilibrium in the face of internal, external and environmental influences. Hyper-stimulation with regards to sexuality can create psychological imbalances and can even be considered as a sex addiction. Lack of proper balance of physiological and psychological processes leads to imbalances in homeostasis.[33]

HORMONAL LEVELS – Refers to level of various hormones that are responsible for the experience of desire, particular sexual desires in the context of current text. See **sex hormones**.

HORNY – feeling or arousing sexual excitement due to external and/or internal stimuli. A slang term referring to built-up sexual desire. There is, generally, a desire to procced further in sexual stimulation.

HRIDAYA GRANTHI – This refers to the "knot of sexual desire" that exist in the "heart." According to various Hindu scriptures, this knot of desire is responsible for deep bondage to worldly life. If this knot is dissolved, then energy begins to flow toward higher consciousness.

HUMAN MICROCOSM – a little world; a world in miniature (opposed to macrocosm); anything that is regarded as a world in miniature: human beings, humanity, society, or the like, viewed as an epitome or miniature version of the world or universe. In the context of experiences of advanced meditators, each human being is considered to be a miniaturized universe. In advanced meditation, it was supposedly discovered that the external reality (i.e. universe) exists within subtle form in each person.[35]

HUMAN SEXUAL RESPONSE CYCLE – is a four-stage model of physiological responses to sexual stimulation, which, in order of their occurrence, are the excitement phase, plateau phase, orgasmic phase, and resolution phase.[36]

HYPER-SEXUALITY – is a proposed clinical diagnosis used by mental healthcare researchers and providers to describe extremely frequent or suddenly increased **libido**.[37]

INDIVIDUALIZED EGO – the "I" or self of any person; a person as thinking, feeling, willing, and distinguishing itself from the selves of others and from objects of its thought.[38]

INFATUATE – to inspire or possess with a foolish or unreasoning passion, as of love, to affect with folly; make foolish or fatuous.[39]

INFATUATION – an intense but short-lived passion or admiration for someone or something.[40]

INNER AWAKENING – This refers to awakening of positive energy and destruction of negative energy. With this awakening of energy, a doorway opens into deeper levels of consciousness to unfold limitless possibilities in one's life.

INNER CHATTERING – This refers to one's self-talk that is generated by the mind while one is awake. This is a process that occurs based on memories, current life circumstances, and thoughts about the future.

INNER ENEMIES – the following six major desire-filled passions of the mind are known as inner enemies: lust, anger, greed, attachment, pride, and envy-jealousy; the negative characteristics of these desire-filled passions prevent man from attaining **moksha** or salvation.

INTELLECT – the power or faculty of the mind by which one knows or understands, as distinguished from that by which one feels and that by which one wills; the understanding component of the mind; the faculty of thinking and acquiring knowledge.[41]

INTERMEDIATE REFRACTORY PERIOD – in the context of the sexual response cycle, this refers to a period of low desire or no desire for further sexual stimulation.

INTERNAL CONFLICTS – refers to conflicts within the internal framework of thoughts, emotions, memories, and desires.

INTRAPSYCHIC CONFLICTS – mental struggles arising from the clash of incompatible or opposing impulses, wishes, drives, or external demands.[42]

INTROSPECTION – The process of looking within oneself and observing as well as deeply perceiving, understanding, and becoming unbiasedly aware of one's inner world.

J. KRISHNAMURTI – a prominent philosopher (1895-1986) who emphasized awareness of one's conditioning as a "pathless path" toward psychological freedom.

KAAM DEV – the Hindu god of human love or desire, often portrayed along with his female counterpart Rati. This is an anthropomorphic form of sex energy.[43]

KARANA SHARIRA – This is the "causal body" that exists in each person. It is a composite of deep impressions that exists within profound depths of one's consciousness. It is also the root of sexual desire and the cause of reincarnation, according to many Eastern spiritual traditions. The word "*karana*" means cause and the word "*sharira*" means body. Hence, this body is much deeper than the physical body (gross body) and the subtle body. The subtle body is a composite of the following: thoughts, emotions, memories, and desires. The causal body (**karana sharira**) is the seed of the subtle and gross body and it originates from ignorance or "nescience" of the one's real self (spirit or **atma**). The term "**jiva**" refers to the spiritual self that is covered by the casual body.

KAREZZA – As its name implies, it comprises of activities like gentle stroking, spooning, skin-to-skin contact, and occasional gentle and non-seminal intercourse.[44]

KEGEL EXERCISES – also known as pelvic floor exercise, consists of repeatedly contracting and relaxing the muscles that form part of the pelvic floor, now sometimes colloquially referred to as the "Kegel muscles."[45]

KEGEL WORKOUTS – repetitive contractions of the pelvic muscles that control the flow in urination in order to strengthen these muscles specially to control or prevent incontinence or to enhance sexual responsiveness during intercourse —called also *Kegels*.[46]

KUNDALINI – refers to a form of primal energy (**shakti**) said to be located at the base of the spine.[47]

LABIDO – Sexual drive. Instinctual psychic energy that in psychoanalytic theory is derived from primitive biological urges (as for sexual pleasure or self-preservation) and is expressed in conscious activity.[48]

LBGTQ – Refers to lesbian, bisexual, gay, transgender, and questioning sexual orientations.[49]

LE PETIT MORT – is an expression which means "the brief loss or weakening of consciousness" and in modern usage refers specifically to "the sensation of orgasm as likened to death." This feeling of weakness or significant reduction of overall energy is experienced, based on hormonal levels and other factors, during the refractory period of the sexual response cycle, particularly in men.[50]

LOW SELF-ESTEEM – this refers to a state of not feeling normal levels of self-esteem where one feels inadequate. In sociology and psychology, self-esteem reflects a person's overall subjective emotional evaluation of his or her own worth. It is a judgment of oneself as well as an attitude toward the self. Self-esteem encompasses beliefs about oneself, (for example, "I am competent", "I am worthy"), as well as emotional states, such as triumph, despair, pride, and shame.[51,52]

LUST – refers to very strong sexual desire.

MANIPURA – is the third primary **chakra** according to yoga tradition. Considered to have 10 petals. These petals correspond to thought waves of spiritual ignorance: thirst, jealousy, treachery, shame, fear, disgust, delusion, foolishness and sadness. [53]

MENTAL HEALTH PROBLEMS – refers to the myriad of problems such as depression, anxiety, bipolar disorder, ADHD, obsessions, compulsions, etc. The DSM – V (Diagnostic and Statistical Manual of Mental Health Disorders) lists mental health diagnoses and related clinical criteria.

MINI-ORGASMIC CURRENT or MINI-ORGASMIC PLEASURE CURRENT – This is the same a **valley orgasm** and refers to the energy that exists within valley orgasms. The presence of a mini-orgasmic current and its rejuvenation occurs when meditation and sexual stimulation are combined together, especially in men. Carefully avoiding the **point- of-no-return** creates the mini-orgasmic current. This is a matter of personal exploration and experience. This term has been created by the author.

MOHANA – This refers to fascination that that occurs in men or women when a beautiful form of the opposite sex is seen.

MOKSHA – is a term in Hinduism and Hindu philosophy which refers to various forms of emancipation, liberation, and release.[54]

MONK – A person who has taken up renunciation from worldly life for the purpose of spiritual upliftment and enlightenment. Also called a "**sadhu**" in Hindu tradition.

MOTIVATION – With regards to sexual stimulation, this refers to "sexual drive." In a more general sense, motivation refers to the reason or reasons one has for acting or behaving in a particular way. It also refers to the general desire or willingness of someone to do something. In the case of sexual stimulation, this refers to the desire to engage in sexual stimulation.

MULADHARA – this is the root chakra that holds potent energy known as **Kundalini**.

MYSTIC – any person who has the capacity to perceive transcendental reality beyond the limitations of conditioned thought.

NADI – energy channels (or nerves) that are perceived in deep meditation. Advanced meditators have identified over 72 thousand such energy nerves. Three main nadis are: Ida, Pingla, Sushumna. Ida (इडा, iḍā "comfort") lies to the left of the spine, whereas pingala (पिङ्गल, piṅgala "tawny (brown)", "golden", "solar") is to the right side of the spine, mirroring the ida. Sushumna (सुषुम्णा, suṣumṇā "very gracious", "kind") runs along the spinal cord in the center, through the seven chakras. Under favorable conditions, the energy of kundalini is said to uncoil and enter sushumna through the *brahma dwara* or gate of Brahma at the base of the spine. The Shiva Samhita, a treatise on yoga states, for example, that out of 350,000 nadis, 14 are particularly important, and among them, the three just mentioned are the three most vital.[55,56]

NEGATIVE RELAXATION – this is a state of relaxation in the refractory period of the sexual response cycle. The level of relaxation is dependent upon the level of intensity of sexual gratification.

NEUROPHYSIOLOGICAL – refers to the physiological (i.e. biological function) processes that are occurring within the brain.

NEUROPHYSIOLOGY – a branch of physiology dealing with the functions of the nervous system. Refers to the function of the brain. Neuroanatomy refers to the structure of the brain.[57]

NIRVANA – state of enlightenment, according to the Buddhist tradition. A state where all disturbances of thought, emotion, memory, and desire have stopped.

NIYAMS – literally means positive duties or observances. Those who are attempting to control sexual impulses follow strict rules (niyams) that regulate sexual activity.

NOCTURNAL EMISSION – "A nocturnal emission, informally known as a wet dream, is a spontaneous orgasm during sleep that includes ejaculation for a male, or vaginal wetness or an orgasm (or both) for a female. Nocturnal emissions are most common during adolescence and early young adult years, but they may happen any time after puberty. It is possible for men to wake up during a wet dream or simply to sleep through it, but for women, some researchers have added the requirement that she should also awaken during the orgasm and perceive that the orgasm happened before it counts as a wet dream. Vaginal lubrication alone does not mean that the female experienced an orgasm.[58]"

NOVELTY – state or quality of being novel, new, or unique; newness. Human mind sees novelty in sexual stimulation and craves, at times, new sexual experiences. Maintaining novelty in a long-term intimate relationship is especially challenging. Hence, there is a need in many couples' lives for meditative stimulation that can maintain novelty using creative approaches.[59]

NYMPHOMANIA – abnormally excessive and uncontrollable sexual desire in women.[60]

ORGASM – is the sudden discharge of accumulated sexual excitement during the sexual response cycle, resulting in rhythmic muscular contractions in the pelvic region characterized by sexual pleasure. Orgasm and ejaculation are two separate physiological processes that are sometimes difficult to distinguish. Orgasm is an intense transient peak sensation of intense pleasure creating an altered state of consciousness associated with reported physical changes.[61, 62]

ORGASMIC ECSTASY – in a general sense, ecstasy is an overpowering emotion or exaltation where there is a state of sudden, intense feeling. Orgasmic ecstasy is a state of orgasmic rejuvenation that abides in one's daily life when proficiency in meditative sexual stimulation occurs. This is a state of transformation from orgasmic pleasure to ecstatic states of euphoria where psychological blocks are naturally removed by transformed sexual energy.[63]

ORGASMIC ENERGY – energy present within the experience of orgasm and energy used to create orgasms. This energy is highly focused, potent, and present in the creation of sexual pleasure.

ORGASMIC INEVITABILITY – as one approaches a sexual peak, the brain triggers a series of reactions where an orgasm is inevitable. This is also known as the "**point-of-no-return**" regarding male orgasm.

ORGASMIC MINI-CURRENTS – these are small orgasmic pleasure currents that flow through the body. The presence of these currents of pleasure is indicative of progress being made in combining meditation with sexual stimulation.

ORGASMIC PLEASURE – the physical and emotional sensation experienced at the peak of sexual excitation, usually resulting from stimulation of the sexual organ and usually accompanied in the male by ejaculation.[64] This can also be experienced in a limited way in the form of pre-orgasmic pleasure.

PARAMHANSA YOGANANDA – A yogi and mystic from India who taught the following: "Self-Realization is the knowing in all parts of body, mind, and soul that you are *now* in possession of the kingdom of God; that you do not have to pray that it come to you; that God's omnipresence is your omnipresence; and that all that you need to do is improve your knowing."[65]

PC MUSCLE – is a hammock-like muscle, found in both sexes, that stretches from the pubic bone to the coccyx (tail bone) forming the floor of the pelvic cavity and supporting the pelvic organs. It is part of the *levator ani* muscle.[66]

PINDA – a Sanskrit name of the human body. Human body is considered to be a miniaturized form of the universe (**brahmanda**).

POINT-OF-NO-RETURN – a state of stimulation where ejaculatory orgasm is inevitable. Same as ejaculatory inevitability.[67]

PRANA – is often referred to as the "life force" or "life energy". It also includes energies present within inanimate objects.[68]

PRE-ORGASMIC MINI-CURRENTS – same as "**mini-orgasmic currents**." These are pleasure currents that can be experienced before entering a full-blown orgasm. The revitalization of these currents is *fundamental* to meditative sexuality.

PSYCHOLOGICAL HOMEOSTASIS – This a term created by the author that refers to the mind (i.e. thought, emotion, memory, and desire) entering and remaining in a state of non-contradiction. It is a state of deep internal interconnection.

PSYCHOLOGICAL TIME – refers to the subjective experience of time, which is measured by one's own perception of the duration of past, current, and future-projection of events. The past and future are creations of thought. Remembrance of the past also occurs in the present and thinking about or planning for the future also occurs in the present. Hence, only the present *actually* exists.[69]

PUBERTY – the condition of being or the period of becoming first capable of reproducing sexually that is brought on by the production of sex hormones and the maturing of the reproductive organs (such as the testes and ovaries). Development of secondary sex characteristics (such as male facial hair growth and female breast development), and in humans and the higher primates, the first occurrence of menstruation in the female. The age at which puberty occurs often construed legally as 14 in boys and 12 in girls.[70]

PUBOCOCCYGEUS MUSCLE – is a hammock-like muscle, found in both sexes, that stretches from the pubic bone to the coccyx (tail bone) forming the floor of the pelvic cavity and supporting the pelvic organs. It is part of the *levator ani* muscle. In simple language, it is the muscle that is used to stop urine from flowing. Strengthening this muscle, especially within men, can provide greater proficiency in pre-orgasmic sexual stimulation.[71]

QUALIA – the internal and subjective component of sense perceptions, arising from stimulation of the senses by external phenomena and internal processes such as dreams. With regards to sexual stimulation, this refers to one's direct and personal experience of sexual pleasure.

REETAS – this refers to raw and refined sex energy that can flow upwards or downwards.

REFRACTORY PERIOD – is usually the recovery phase after orgasm during which it is physiologically impossible for a man to have additional orgasms due to increase in the penile sensory threshold.[72]

RESOLUTION STAGE – in women, the vagina begins a series of regular contractions; in the man, the penis also contracts rhythmically to expel the sperm and semen.[73]

RETICULAR ACTIVATION SYSTEM – this part of the brain plays a major part in sexual arousal.

SADHAKA – a person who follows a particular *sādhanā*, or a way of life designed to realize the goal of one's ultimate ideal, whether it is merging with one's eternal Source, *brahman*, or realization of one's personal deity.[74]

SADHANA – refers to a multitude of spiritual practices that are aimed at opening the door into spiritual reality. The word "**sadhaka**" refers to one who is performing "**sadhana**" to reach "siddhi." Siddhi is a state of attainment of spiritual powers. The apex of spiritual practices is known as "Samadhi" where the polarity of the mind is transcended.

SADHU – a person who has taken special vows and has left worldly life for spiritual realization. There are many Hindu organizations that have "sadhus" who follow strict rules and perform deep meditation practices. In Western religious traditions, there are similar individual who have dedicated themselves totally toward higher realization.

SAGE – one (such as a profound philosopher) distinguished for wisdom. Also refers to a mature or venerable man of sound judgment.[75]

SAHASRARA – is generally considered the seventh primary chakra according to yoga traditions. This is a 1000 petal spiritual lotus that exists at the top of the head. Once opened through a multitude of psycho-spiritual practices, one enters into a state of enlightenment.[76]

SAMSKARA (or SANSKARA) – these are mental impressions, recollections, and psychological imprints that remain in the mind that have the propensity to *generate* desire based on past experiences.

SANSKRIT – is the primary liturgical language of Hinduism; There are many mantras (sound vibrations) that are in this language that have various psychological effects when chanted regularly.[77]

SAT-CHIT-ANANDA – representing "existence, consciousness, and bliss" or "truth, consciousness, and bliss solidified." An epithet and description for the subjective experience of the ultimate, unchanging reality in Hinduism called Brahman (i.e. God).[78]

SATIATION – with regards to sexual stimulation, this refers to a state of deep satisfaction of desire where there is no further desire.[79]

SATTVIKA INTELLIGENCE – a level of awakened intelligence where sexual passion is in a transformative process moving toward ecstasy. Sattvika refers to a mode of mental functioning where there is significant reduction in overall desire for stimulation. Beyond the state of "sattvika" is a state of uninterrupted pure joy (**ananda**).

SELF – refers to one's one existence.

SELF-ESTEEM – respect for or pride about oneself.[80]

SELF IMAGE – The conception that one has of oneself, including an assessment of qualities and personal worth.[81]

SELF-WORTH – refers to one's evaluation of oneself.[82]

SEMEN – is an organic fluid that may contain spermatozoa. It is secreted by the gonads (sexual glands) and other sexual organs of male or hermaphroditic animals and can fertilize female ova. Semen is only one percent sperm; the rest is composed of over 200 separate proteins, as well as vitamins and minerals including vitamin C, calcium, chlorine, citric acid, fructose, lactic acid, magnesium, nitrogen, phosphorus, potassium, sodium, vitamin B12, and zinc.[83]

SEX – either of the two major forms of individuals that occur in many species and that are distinguished respectively as female or male especially on the basis of their reproductive organs and structures. The sum of the structural, functional, and behavioral characteristics of organisms that are involved in reproduction marked by the union of gametes and that distinguish males and females. This can also refer to the act of sexual stimulation as in "having sex."[84]

SEX ENERGY – refers to neuropsychological energy that is used in creating orgasmic experiences.

SEX ENERGY SUBLIMATION – refers to the process of conserving sex energy for greater purposes in life. This energy is eventually stored in the brain and is available for use in multiple areas in one's life.

SEX HORMONES – refers to biological levels of key sex hormones. Sexual reproduction motivation is influenced by hormones such as testosterone, estrogen, progesterone, oxytocin, and vasopressin. In most mammalian species, sex hormones control the ability to engage in sexual behaviors. However, sex hormones do not directly regulate the ability to copulate in primates (including humans). Rather, sex hormones in primates are only one influence on the motivation to engage in sexual behaviors.[34]

SEX KNOT (GRANTHI) DISSOLUTION CYCLE – refers to the process of transcending the deep psychological "knot" of sexual desire for the purpose of inward awakening (spiritual awakening). The dissolution of the sex knot can potentially lead to the awakening of the non-mechanical, non-repetitive, non-fragmentary aspects of the mind. (This idea of awaking of non-mechanical parts of the brain has been discussed by **J. Krishnamurti**.)

SEX/ORGASM/CELIBACY CONTINUUM – this refers to the flow of sexual energy among two poles: one is whole body orgasm and the other is **brahmacharya** (celibacy).

SEXUAL APPETITE – refers to the appetite or physical and psychological demand for sexual stimulation as per one's desires.

SEXUAL AROUSAL – the arousal of sexual desire, during, or, in anticipation of sexual activity. Arousal is the activation of desire for sexual stimulation. Colloquially, this is known as "getting turned on. "A number of physiological responses occur in the body and mind as preparation for sexual intercourse, and these responses continue to expand and modify as excitation increases. Genital responses are not the only changes, yet they are noticeable and necessary for consensual and comfortable intercourse.[85]

SEXUAL ATTRACTION – refers to an attractive response in the mind of an individual toward another person(s) who is perceived as attractive.

SEXUAL CONTINENCE – is a form of sexual intercourse in which the penetrative partner does not attempt to ejaculate within the receptive partner, but instead attempts to remain in the plateau phase of intercourse for as long as possible, avoiding seminal emission.[86]

SEXUAL DESIRE – is a motivational state and an interest in "sexual objects or activities, or as a wish, need or drive to seek out sexual objects or to engage in sexual activities.[87]

SEXUAL ENERGY – refers to the flow of energy that exist within the entire sexual response cycle.

SEXUAL ESSENCES – refers to refined sex energy currents that contained transmuted sex energy.

SEXUAL FANTASY – mental images of an erotic nature that can lead to sexual arousal.[88]

SEXUAL INTERCOURSE – principally the insertion and thrusting of the penis, usually when erect, into the vagina for sexual pleasure, reproduction, or both. This is also known as vaginal intercourse or vaginal sex.[89]

SEXUAL ORIENTATION – is an enduring pattern of romantic or sexual attraction (or a combination of these) to persons of the opposite sex or gender, the same sex or gender, or to both sexes or more than one gender.[90]

SHAKTI – meaning "power" and is the primordial cosmic energy which comprises of dynamic forces that are thought to move through the entire universe.[91] Shakti is the sex energy in its various forms.

SHIVA – the word "Shivam" in **Sanskrit** means all the following: consciousness, auspiciousness, and life force. Shiva refers to destruction of negativity and creation of positive states of mind.

SHIVA LINGAM – is an abstract or aniconic representation of the Hindu deity, Shiva, used for worship in temples, smaller shrines, or as self-manifested natural objects. It represents the absolute oneness of male and female energies.[92]

SHIVA SUTRAS – these are 114 Sanskrit verses that describe various meditation techniques. One of these key verses is: "At the start of sexual union, keep attention to the fire in the beginning, and so continuing, avoid the embers toward the end."

SOSHANA – this is a state of intense attraction that causes the semen in the male body to start moving. It is a "churning" of subtle neuropsychological energy. Semen is created by this "churning" process. Semen exists in subtle form throughout the male body and the attractive response creates a state of psychological and physiological emaciation where energy is pulled from other areas of the physical body and the mind.

SOUL – refers to the non-physical aspect of oneself. It is due to the presence of the spiritual spark that mental abilities are possible. Mental abilities such as reason, character, feeling, consciousness, memory, perception, thinking, etc. are cognized due to the existence of the "spiritual observer" which is the witnessing consciousness. The Sanskrit word for "soul" is "**atma**."[93]

STAMBHANA – This refers to stupefaction that arrests one's attention. Stupefaction is a state of bafflement, perplexity, and befuddlement with respect to sexual arousal. It is a state where the mind's functions get focused or concentrated on a person who appears highly attractive.

SUBCONSCIOUS MIND – part of one's overall consciousness that is not currently in focal awareness.[94]

SUBJECTIVE EXAMINATION – this refers to one's own inner exploration of mental and emotional processes and experiences in the context of sexual attraction, sexual arousal, and sexual stimulation.

SUBLIMATION – this refers to the upward follow of sex energy without the problems of suppression or hyper-indulgence due to suppression.

SUPPRESSION – refers to forcefully controlling sexually impulses. Suppression generally has a "spring like" action that eventually leads to heavy indulgence, particularly with regards to sexual pleasure.

SUTRA – is a **Sanskrit** word that means "string" or "thread" where deep meaning is hidden within a small phrase. The Yoga Sutras of Patanjali are famous around the world for such hidden meaning.[95]

SWADHISTANA (SEX ENERGY CHAKRA) – is the second primary chakra in the 7-chakra system. It is considered to be location of immense sex energy.

TANTRA – this word simply means to "weave together" broken emotions, energies, and thoughts in to a whole.

TANTRIC YOGI – an individual who combines sexual stimulation with meditation for the purpose of integrating sexual energies.

TAO – is a metaphysical concept in the Chinese tradition stating the that all reality is ONE.

TAOIST SEXUAL PRACTICES – specific practices in the Taoist tradition about combining meditation with sexual stimulation.

TAPANA – refers to burning and inflaming of the emotional heart that occurs if there is rejection. Such rejection from a potential mate that causes emotional pain (i.e. emotional burning) and heartache.

TRANSFORMATION - a thorough or dramatic change in the inner form and function of sex energy.

TRANSMUTATION – the action of changing raw sex energy into highly refined and beneficial forms.

ULTIMATE REALITY – refers to the substratum (i.e. God, Brahman, etc.) upon which the world of names and forms appears.

UNMADANA – This refers to "intoxication" where a person is deeply absorbed in the form of the other person. It is a state of psychological fixation and inner "intoxication" where one's senses are drawn deeply into the form of another person who is perceived to be attractive.

URDHVA – is a **Sanskrit** term meaning "up" or "upward."

URDHVAREETA – refers to the upward flow of sex energy.

URDHVA-REETA BRAHMACHARAYA – refers to the upward flow of sex energy without frictional orgasm so that the entire sex energy is sublimated and transmuted.

VALLEY ORGASMS – these are mini-orgasms that appear as one relaxes within oneself after significant stimulation. The orgasms are pre-orgasmic and have the **mini-orgasmic pleasure current** (energy flow) within them.

VASANA – the desire to experience pleasure due to past memories of pleasurable experiences or desire to experience pleasure that has not yet been experienced. This is a **Sanskrit** term used to describe deep-seated desires that generally have a cyclical nature.

VASOCONGESTION – is the swelling of bodily tissues caused by increased vascular blood flow and a localized increase in blood pressure. Typical causes of vasocongestion in humans includes menstruation, sexual arousal, REM sleep, strong emotions, illnesses and allergic reactions.[96]

VEERAYA – **Sanskrit** word for "semen."

VIJNANBHAIRAV TANTRA – this is a **Sanskrit** text that shows 114 meditation techniques. A key technique with regards to sexuality is as follows: "At the start of sexual union, keep attention to the fire in the beginning and so continuing, avoid the embers toward the end."

VISHUDDHI (THROAT CHAKRA) – is the fifth primary chakra (energy center). Sex energy sublimated to the level of this chakra unleashes an unlimited feeling of happiness and freedom that allows abilities and skills to blossom. Along with this stage of development there is deep clarity within one's voice, a talent for singing and speech also develops, as well as balanced and calm thoughts.

VRUTTI – is a technical term in yoga meant to indicate that the contents of mental awareness are disturbances in the medium of consciousness. Just as the ocean has waves, the mind (i.e. thoughts, emotions, memories, and desires) are like waves on the substratum of consciousness. Consciousness can be considered to be: God, Spirit, Truth, Bliss, etc.[97]

WHOLE BODY ORGASM – an intense orgasm that is felt throughout the body. It is an experience of intense sexual pleasure.

YANG - (in Chinese philosophy) the active male principle of the universe, characterized as male and creative and associated with heaven, heat, and light.

YIN - (in Chinese philosophy) the passive female principle of the universe, characterized as female and sustaining and associated with earth, dark, and cold.

YOGA – to connect or join with one's inner and/or higher power (God, Brahman, etc.)

YOGI – A practitioner of yoga.

YOG NIDRA – is a state of consciousness between waking and sleeping, like the "going-to-sleep" stage. It is a state in which the body is completely relaxed, and the practitioner becomes systematically and increasingly aware of the inner world within oneself due to the stopping of the mind's projection system.[98]

YOGIC MASTERS – teachers of yoga using multiple approaches.

NOTES & REFERENCES

CHAPTER ONE

[A] (n.d.). Retrieved from http://www.brainyquote.com/quotes/authors/p/plato.html

[1] In the opinion of the author, heavy losses of sexual fluids in men causes decreased overall orgasmic energy, which is essential or fundamental energy existing in each organ of the body. The sex act uses(?) this orgasmic energy, which exists in subtle form in and is extracted from each organ in the body, especially the brain. Hence, the psychic or spiritual energy known as **ojas** that could potentially be stored does not get stored. Suffice it to say, the negative relaxation felt after ejaculating is called "negative" by the author because a heavy price has been paid for this relaxation, due to the concurrent, tremendous loss of spiritual energy known as **prana. Prana** is the divine power that is responsible for creating experiences within the waking and dream states. **Prana** decreases substantially when ejaculation occurs, and this causes the mind to dip down into lower levels of consciousness. This is one of the main reasons why celibacy is strongly advocated by many traditional spiritual paths in many religions.

CHAPTER TWO

[1] Desire Quotes. (n.d.). Retrieved July 21, 2017, from https://www.brainyquote.com/quotes/keywords/desire.html

[2.3.4.5.6] Sexual Response Cycle. (2010). In Encyclopedia Britannica. Retrieved March 10, 2010, from Encyclopedia Britannica Online: http://www.britannica.com/Ebchecked/topic/537200/sexual-response-cycle

[7,8] Mah, K. & Binik, Y.M. "The Nature of Human Orgasm: A Critical Review of Major Trends" *Clinical Psychology Review*. Volume 21, Number 6 (2001): 823-856.

[9, 10] Sexual Response Cycle. (2010). In Encyclopedia Britannica. Retrieved March 10, 2010, from Encyclopedia Britannica Online: http://www.britannica.com/Ebchecked/topic/537200/sexual-response-cycle

CHAPTER THREE

[1] Kandel, E. R. (1999). Biology and the future of psychoanalysis: A new intellectual framework for psychiatry revisited. American Journal of Psychiatry, 156, 505–524.

[2] Dennett, D. ''Quining Qualia''". Ase.tufts.edu. 1985-11-21. Retrieved 2010-12-03. https://sites.google.com/site/minddict/q

[3] Levine, S. B. (2003). "The nature of sexual desire: A clinician's perspective". Archives of Sexual Behavior. 32 (3): 279–285. PMID 12807300. Doi:10.1023/A:1023421819465.

[4] Gonzaga, G. C.; Turner, R. A.; Keltner, D.; Campos, B.; Altemus, M. (2006). "Romantic Love and Sexual Desire in Close Relationships". Emotion. 6 (2): 163–179. PMID 16768550. Doi:10.1037/1528-3542.6.2.163.

CHAPTER FOUR

[1] Mosby's Medical, Nursing and Allied Health Dictionary, Fourth Edition, Mosby-Year Book Inc., 1994, p. 335

[2] Blood. (2017, July 21). Retrieved July 21, 2017, from https://www.merriam-webster.com/dictionary/blood

[3] Bones. (2017, July 18). Retrieved July 21, 2017, from http://en.wikipedia.org/wiki/Bones

[4] Birbrair, Alexander; Frenette, Paul S. (2016-03-01). "Niche heterogeneity in the bone marrow". *Annals of the New York Academy of Sciences*. 1370: 82–96. ISSN 1749-6632. PMC 4938003 Freely accessible. PMID 27015419. doi:10.1111/nyas.13016

[5] Brahmacharya.info. (n.d.). Retrieved July 21, 2017, from http://www.brahmacharya.info/

[6] Benefits of celibacy: Why Practice Celibacy (Brahmacharya)? From: https://www.youtube.com/watch?v=9hZzYFWbcsw&t=114s

CHAPTER FIVE

[1] mind - definition of mind in English | Oxford Dictionaries". Oxford Dictionaries | English. Retrieved 2017-05-08. [2] How Big Is Porn? (2001, May 25). Retrieved July 23, 2017, from https://www.forbes.com/2001/05/25/0524porn.html

[3] Atavism. (n.d.). Retrieved July 23, 2017, from http://www.dictionary.com/browse/atavism

[4] Wilson, Gary. Your Brain on Porn: Internet Pornography and the Emerging Science of Addiction (Kindle Locations 167-176). Commonwealth Publishing. Kindle Edition.

[5] Wilson, Gary. Your Brain on Porn: Internet Pornography and the Emerging Science of Addiction (Kindle Locations 177-181). Commonwealth Publishing. Kindle Edition.

[6] Valerie Voon, et al., "Neural Correlates of Sexual Cue Reactivity in Individuals with and without Compulsive Sexual Behaviours", *PLOS One* (2014): DOI: 10.1371/ journal.pone. 0102419.

[7] Wilson, Gary. Your Brain on Porn: Internet Pornography and the Emerging Science of Addiction (Kindle Locations 2840-2843). Commonwealth Publishing. Kindle Edition.

CHAPTER SIX

[1] White, David Gordon (ed.) (2000). *Tantra in Practice. Princeton University Press. P. 9. ISBN 0-691-05779-6.*

[2] http://philosiblog.com/2011/09/05/your-vision-will-become-clear-only-when-you-can-look-into-your-own-heart-who-looks-outside-dreams-who-looks-inside-awakes/

CHAPTER SEVEN

[1] http://www.biggerloads.com/penis-size/kegels-men.html
[2] http://www.wikihow.com/Do-PC-Muscle-Exercises
[3] http://www.healthline.com/health-slideshow/kegel-exercises-for-men
[4] http://www.health24.com/Sex/Problems/Sexual-superhero-PC-muscle-exercise-20120721
[5] Vern L. Bulloch, *Science in the Bedroom*, 1994
[6] azmajian, Richard V. (1967). "The Influence of Testicular Sensory Stimuli on the Dream". *Journal of the American Psychoanalytic Association*. 15 (1): 83–98. PMID 6032147. doi:10.1177/000306516701500103

CHAPTER EIGHT

[1] Cabanac, Michel (2002). "What is emotion?" *Behavioural Processes* 60(2): 69-83.

CHAPTER NINE

[1] Swami Sivananda Quotes. (n.d.). Retrieved July 21, 2017, from https://www.brainyquote.com/quotes/quotes/s/swamisivan165766.html

[2] Guru Quotes -. (2017, June 10). Retrieved July 21, 2017, from http://shivyogindia.com/guru-quotes-19/

GLOSSARY

[1] "Encyclopædia Britannica Online, "Adultery"". Britannica.com. Retrieved 2010-07-12

[2] "The Ancient Powerful Practices of Hindu Meditation". *The Way of Meditation*. 2015-05-05. Retrieved 2017-03-31.

[3] Williams, Raymond (2001). *Introduction to Swaminarayan Hinduism*. Cambridge: Cambridge University Press. p. 83. ISBN 0 521 65279 0.

[4] Crowe, LC; George, WH (1989). "Alcohol and human sexuality: Review and integration". Psychological Bulletin. 105 (3): 374–86. PMID 2660179. doi:10.1037/0033-2909.105.3.374

[5] *Carey, Francis*. Organic Chemistry *(4 ed.)*. ISBN 0072905018. *Retrieved 5 February 2013.*

[6] Ananda-What is Ananda?-Definition of the Sanskrit Word. (n.d.). Retrieved July 05, 2017, from https://www.ananda.org/yogapedia/ananda/

[7] Woodroffe, J. *The Serpent Power* – Dover Publications, New York, 1974 p. 120

[8] Arousal. (2017, June 17). Retrieved June 20, 2017, from https://en.wikipedia.org/wiki/Arousal

[9] Atavism. (n.d.). Retrieved July 23, 2017, from http://www.dictionary.com/browse/atavism

[10] John Bowker (2000), The Concise Oxford Dictionary of World Religions, Oxford University Press, ISBN 978-0192800947

[11] Swami Ranganathananda (1991). Human Being in Depth: A Scientific Approach to Religion. SUNY Press. p. 21. ISBN 0791406792.

[12] The Franklin Institute Inc. "Blood – The Human Heart". Archived from the original on 5 March 2009. Retrieved 19 March 2009.

[13] Fergusson, Rosalind; Eric Partridge; Paul Beale (December 1993). Shorter Slang Dictionary. Routledge. p. 21. ISBN 978-0-415-08866-4.

[14] Schmidt, Richard F.; Lang, Florian; Heckmann, Manfred (2010-11-30). "What are the organs of the immune system?". © IQWiG (Institute for Quality and Efficiency in Health Care): 3/7

[15] Brahmachari. (n.d.). Retrieved June 20, 2017, from http://www.dictionary.com/browse/brahmachari

[16] James Lochtefeld, "Brahmacharya" in The Illustrated Encyclopedia of Hinduism, Vol. 1: A–M, pp. 120, Rosen Publishing. ISBN 9780823931798

[17] John A. Grimes (1996). A Concise Dictionary of Indian Philosophy: Sanskrit Terms Defined in English. State University of New York Press. pp. 100–101. ISBN 978-0-7914-3067-5.

[18] Mosby's Medical, Nursing and Allied Health Dictionary, Fourth Edition, Mosby-Year Book Inc., 1994, p. 335

[19] Coitus. (n.d.). Retrieved June 21, 2017, from https://www.merriam-webster.com/dictionary/coitus

[20] Watts, Alan W. (1970). Nature, Man and Woman. Random House Inc. Vintage Books Edition. p. 172. LCCN 58-8266.

[21] Conscious mind. (n.d.). Retrieved June 21, 2017, from http://www.thefreedictionary.com/Conscious mind

[22] Dhatu. (2017, June 15). Retrieved June 21, 2017, from https://en.wikipedia.org/wiki/Dhatu

[23] Sanskrit-English Dictionary by Monier-Williams, (c) 1899

[24] (n.d.). The Gerson Institute of Ayurvedic Medicine. Retrieved July 18, 2017, from http://ayurveda.md/component/content/article?id=67&Itemid=9

[25] Ejaculate. (n.d.). Retrieved June 21, 2017, from http://www.dictionary.com/browse/ejaculate

[26] Ejaculation. (n.d.). Retrieved June 21, 2017, from http://www.dictionary.com/browse/ejaculation?s=t

[27] Ejaculatory inevitability. (n.d.). Retrieved June 21, 2017, from http://www.urbandictionary.com/define.php?term=ejaculatory inevitability

[28] The Editors of Encyclopædia Britannica. (2015, January 30). Sexual intercourse. Retrieved June 21, 2017, from https://www.britannica.com/science/sexual-intercourse#ref264522

[29] Block, Susan (27 February 2005). "All About Female Ejaculation". Counterpunch. Archived from the original on 23 March 2010. Retrieved 4 February 2010.

[30] Brosius, J (2009), "The Fragmented Gene", Annals of the New York Academy of Sciences, 1178: 186–193, doi:10.1111/j.1749-6632.2009.05004.x

[31] Attridge, Harold. W., and R. A. Oden, Jr. (1981), Philo of Byblos: The Phoenician History: Introduction, Critical Text, Translation, Notes, CBQMS 9 (Washington: D. C.: The Catholic Biblical Association of America).

[32] Zorea, Aharon (2014). Steroids (Health and Medical Issues Today). Westport, CT: Greenwood Press. p. 10. ISBN 978-1440802997.

[33] What is a homeostatic imbalance? | Socratic. (n.d.). Retrieved June 20, 2017, from https://socratic.org/questions/what-is-a-homeostatic-imbalance

[34] Wallen K (2001). "Sex and context: hormones and primate sexual motivation.". *Hormone Behaviour*. **40** (2): 339–357. PMID 11534996. doi:10.1006/hbeh.2001.1696 (changed type size/font to match rest)

[35] Microcosm. (n.d.). Retrieved June 20, 2017, from http://www.dictionary.com/browse/microcosm

[36] John Archer, Barbara Lloyd (2002). Sex and Gender. Cambridge University Press. pp. 85–88. ISBN 0521635330. Retrieved August 25, 2012

[37] Stein, D. J. (2008). Classifying hypersexual disorders: Compulsive, impulsive, and addictive models. Psychiatric Clinics of North America, 31, 587–592.

[38] Ego. (n.d.). Retrieved June 19, 2017, from http://www.dictionary.com/browse/ego

[39] Infatuate. (n.d.). Retrieved June 19, 2017, from http://www.dictionary.com/browse/infatuate?s=t

[40] Infatuation. (n.d.). Retrieved June 19, 2017, from http://www.dictionary.com/browse/infatuation?s=t

[41] Intellect. (n.d.). Retrieved June 19, 2017, from http://www.dictionary.com/browse/intellect?s=ts

[42] Intrapsychic conflict. (n.d.). Retrieved June 19, 2017, from http://medical-dictionary.thefreedictionary.com / intrapsychic conflict

[43] Kāṇe, Pāṇḍuraṅga Vāmana; Institute, Bhandarkar Oriental Research (1958). History of Dharmaśāstra

[44] Karezza. (n.d.). Retrieved June 20, 2017, from http://www.sacred-texts.com/sex/krz/krz04.htm

[45] Bridgeman, Bruce; Roberts, Steven G. (2010-03-01). "The 4-3-2 method for Kegel exercises". American Journal of Men's Health. 4 (1): 75–76. ISSN 1557-9891. PMID 19477754. doi:10.1177/1557988309331798

[46] Kegel Exercises. (n.d.). Retrieved June 19, 2017, from https://www.merriam-webster.com/dictionary/Kegel%20exercises

[47] Greer, John Michael (2003). The New Encyclopedia of the Occult (1st ed.). St. Paul, Minnesota: Llewellyn Publications. p. 262. ISBN 9781567183368.

[48] Labido. (n.d.). Retrieved June 19, 2017, from http://www.urbandictionary.com/define.php?term=Labido

[49] LBGTQ. (n.d.). Retrieved June 19, 2017, from http://acronyms.thefreedictionary.com/LBGTQ

[50] Vaitl, D.; Birbaumer, N.; Gruzelier, J.; Jamieson, G. A.; Kotchoubey, B.; Kübler, A.; Lehmann, D.; Miltner, W. H.; et al. (2005). "Psychobiology of Altered States of Consciousness". Psychological Bulletin. 131 (1): 98–127. PMID 15631555. doi:10.1037/0033-2909.131.1.98

[51] Hewitt, John P. (2009). Oxford Handbook of Positive Psychology. Oxford University Press. Pp. 217–224. ISBN 978-0-19-518724-3.

[52] Hewitt, John P. (2009). Oxford Handbook of Positive Psychology. Oxford University Press. pp. 217–224. ISBN 978-0-19-518724-3.

[53] Solis, Michael (2011-11-29). Balancing the Chakras. Charles River Editors. ISBN 9781619828780.

[54] John Bowker, The Oxford Dictionary of World Religions, Oxford University Press, ISBN 978-0192139658, pp. 650

[55] Chakras and Nadis. (n.d.). Retrieved June 19, 2017, from http://www.maliniyoga.com/en/chakras-and-nadis/

[56] McEvilley, Thomas. "The Spinal Serpent", in: Harper and Brown, p.94.

[57] Neurophysiology. (n.d.). Retrieved July 04, 2017, from http://www.dictionary.com/browse/neurophysiological

[58] Meng, X; Fan, L; Liu, J; Wang, T; Yang, J; Wang, J; Wang, S; Ye, Z (2013). "Fresh semen quality in ejaculates produced by nocturnal emission in men with idiopathic anejaculation". Fertility and Sterility. 100 (5): 1248–52. PMID 23987518. doi:10.1016/j.fertnstert.2013.07.1979.

[59] "Novelty." Dictionary.com. Dictionary.com, n.d. Web. 30 June 2017.

[60] "Nymphomania." Dictionary.com. Dictionary.com, n.d. Web. 28 June 2017.

[61] Masters, William H.; Johnson, Virginia E.; Reproductive Biology Research Foundation (U.S.) (1966). Human Sexual Response. Little, Brown. p. 366. ISBN 0-316-54987-8.
[62] Alwaal, A. (2015, November). Normal male sexual function: emphasis on orgasm and ejaculation. Retrieved July 19, 2017, from https://www.ncbi.nlm.nih.gov/pmc/articles/PMC4896089/pdf/nihms-789951.pdf

[63] Ecstasy. (n.d.). Retrieved July 03, 2017, from http://www.dictionary.com/browse/ecstasy

[64] Orgasm. (n.d.). Retrieved July 04, 2017, from http://www.dictionary.com/browse/orgasmic

[65] Paramhansa Yogananda (1893-1952): His life, books, teachings, and more... (n.d.). Retrieved July 05, 2017, from https://www.ananda.org/about-ananda-sangha/lineage/paramhansa-yogananda/

[66] Essential Clinical Anatomy. K.L. Moore & A.M. Agur. Lippincott, 2nd ed. 2002. Page 217

[67] Harvey, 1925, 154-155; U Kala II p. 173, ch. 168

[68] Swami Satyananda Saraswati (September 1981). "Prana: the Universal Life Force". Yogamag.net. Bihar School of Yoga. Retrieved 31 July 2015.

[69] Evans V (2013). Language and time: a cognitive linguistics approach. Cambridge: Cambridge University Press. ISBN 978-1-107-04380-0.

[70] Puberty. (n.d.). Retrieved July 01, 2017, from https://www.merriam-webster.com/dictionary/puberty

[71] Wallner C, Maas C, Dabhoiwala N, Lamers W, Deruiter M (2006). "Evidence for the innervation of the puborectalis muscle by the levator ani nerve". Neurogastroenterol Motil. 18 (12): 1121–1122. PMID 17109696. doi:10.1111/j.1365-2982.2006.00846.x

[72] Ross Morrow (2013). Sex Research and Sex Therapy: A Sociological Analysis of Masters and Johnson. Routledge. p. 91. ISBN 1134134657. Retrieved September 9, 2016.

[73] Resolution stage. (n.d.). Retrieved July 01, 2017, from https://www.britannica.com/topic/resolution-stage

[74] Klostermaier, Klaus K. (1994). A survey of Hinduism. SUNY Press. p. 346. ISBN 978-0-7914-2109-3.

[75] Sage. (n.d.). Retrieved July 19, 2017, from https://www.merriam-webster.com/dictionary/sage

[76] "The Sahasrara Chakra". Kheper. Retrieved May 15, 2014.

[77] Uta Reinöhl (2016). Grammaticalization and the Rise of Configurationality in Indo-Aryan. Oxford University Press. pp. xiv, 1–16. ISBN 978-0-19-873666-0.

[78] Gurajada Suryanarayana Murty (2002), Paratattvagaṇṇitadarśanam, Motilal Banarsidass, ISBN 978-8120818217, page 303

[79] Satiate. (n.d.). Retrieved July 01, 2017, from http://www.dictionary.com/browse/satiation

[80] "Self-esteem." The Free Dictionary. Farlex, n.d. Web. 30 June 2017.

[81] "Self-image." The Free Dictionary. Farlex, n.d. Web. 30 June 2017.

[82] "Self-worth." The Free Dictionary. Farlex, n.d. Web. 30 June 2017.

[83] Mann, T (1954). "The Biochemistry of Semen". London: Methuen & Co; New York: John Wiley & Sons. Retrieved November 9, 2013.

[84] Sex. (n.d.). Retrieved July 04, 2017, from https://www.merriam-webster.com/dictionary/sex

[85] "Your introduction to foreplay". Archived from the original on 2007-06-18. Retrieved 2007-05-18.

[86] Watts, Alan W. (1970). Nature, Man and Woman. Random House Inc. Vintage Books Edition. p. 172. LCCN 58-8266.

[87] Regan, P.C.; Atkins, L. (2006). "Sex Differences and Similarities in Frequency and Intensity of Sexual Desire". Social Behavior & Personality: An International Journal. 34 (1): 95–101. doi:10.2224/sbp.2006.34.1.95

[88] "Sexual fantasy." The Free Dictionary. Farlex, n.d. Web. 29 June 2017.

[89] Keath Roberts (2006). Sex. Lotus Press. p. 145. ISBN 8189093592. Retrieved August 17, 2012.

[90] "Sexual orientation, homosexuality and bisexuality". American Psychological Association. Archived from the original on August 8, 2013. Retrieved August 10, 2013.

[91] Insoll, Professor of African and Islamic Archaeology Timothy; Insoll, Timothy (2002-09-11). Archaeology and World Religion. Routledge. p. 36. ISBN 9781134597987.

[92] Johnson, W.J. (2009). A dictionary of Hinduism (1st ed.). Oxford: Oxford University Press. ISBN 9780191726705. Retrieved 5 January 2016.

[93] "Soul (noun) - Oxford English Dictional (online full edition)". Oxford English Dictionary (OED). Oxford English Dictional (OED). Retrieved 1 December 2016.

[94] A Dictionary of Psychology Andrew M. Colman. Oxford University Press, 2006. Oxford Reference Online. Oxford University Press. King's College London.

[95] M Winternitz (2010 Reprint), A History of Indian Literature, Volume 1, Motilal Banarsidass, ISBN 978-81-208-0264-3, pages 249

[96] Vern L. Bulloch, Science in the Bedroom, 1994 .

[97] I.K. Taimni, The Science of Yoga: The Yoga-Sutras of Patanjali in Sanskrit , ISBN 978-81-7059-211-2

[98] Rama, Swami. Mandukya Upanishad: Enlightenment Without God. ISBN 0-89389-084-7.

INDEX

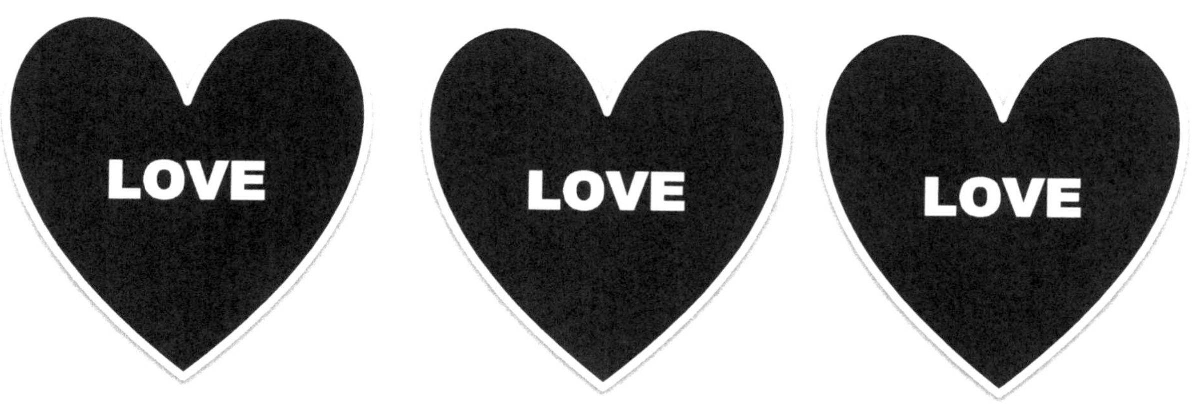
LOVE
LOVE
LOVE